Dental Biomaterials

Editors

JACK L. FERRACANE
CARMEM S. PFEIFER
LUIZ E. BERTASSONI

DENTAL CLINICS OF NORTH AMERICA

www.dental.theclinics.com

October 2022 • Volume 66 • Number 4

ELSEVIER

1600 John F. Kennedy Boulevard • Suite 1800 • Philadelphia, Pennsylvania, 19103-2899

http://www.dental.theclinics.com

DENTAL CLINICS OF NORTH AMERICA Volume 66, Number 4
October 2022 ISSN 0011-8532, ISBN: 978-0-323-84896-1

Editor: John Vassallo; j.vassallo@elsevier.com
Developmental Editor: Ann Gielou M. Posedio

Dental Clinics of North America (ISSN 0011-8532) is published quarterly by Elsevier Inc., 360 Park Avenue South, New York, NY 10010-1710. Months of issue are January, April, July, and October. Business and Editorial Offices: 1600 John F. Kennedy Boulevard, Suite 1800, Philadelphia, PA 19103-2899. Periodicals postage paid at New York, NY and additional mailing offices. Subscription prices are $323.00 per year (domestic individuals), $854.00 per year (domestic institutions), $100.00 per year (domestic students/residents), $377.00 per year (Canadian individuals), $863.00 per year (Canadian institutions), $100.00 per year (Canadian students/residents) $441.00 per year (international individuals), $863.00 per year (international institutions), and $200.00 per year (international students/residents). International air speed delivery is included in all *Clinics* subscription prices. All prices are subject to change without notice. **POSTMASTER:** Send address changes to *Dental Clinics of North America*, Elsevier Health Sciences Division, Subscription Customer Service, 3251 Riverport Lane, Maryland Heights, MO 63043. **Customer Service (orders, claims, online, change of address): Elsevier Health Sciences Division, Subscription Customer Service, 3251 Riverport Lane, Maryland Heights, MO 63043. Tel: 1-800-654-2452 (U.S. and Canada). Fax: 314-447-8029. E-mail: journalscustomerservice-usa@elsevier.com (for print support); journalsonlinesupport-usa@elsevier. com (for online support).**

Reprints. For copies of 100 or more, of articles in this publication, please contact the Commercial Reprints Department, Elsevier Inc., 360 Park Avenue South, New York, NY 10010-1710. Tel.: 212-633-3874; Fax: 212-633-3820; E-mail: reprints@elsevier.com.

The Dental Clinics of North America is covered in *MEDLINE/PubMed (Index Medicus), Current Contents/Clinical Medicine, ISI/BIOMED* and *Clinahl.*

Contributors

EDITORS

JACK L. FERRACANE, PhD
Professor and Chair, Department of Restorative Dentistry, Oregon Health & Science University, Portland, Oregon, USA

CARMEM S. PFEIFER, DDS, PhD
Professor and Division Director of Biomaterials and Biomechanics, Department of Restorative Dentistry, Oregon Health & Science University, Portland, Oregon, USA

LUIZ E. BERTASSONI, DDS, PhD
Associate Professor, Department of Restorative Dentistry, Oregon Health & Science University, Portland, Oregon, USA

AUTHORS

AMIRAH ALAMMAR, BDS
Sijam Medical Center, Alghadeer District, Riyadh, Saudi Arabia

HONGSEOK AN, DDS, MSD
Restorative Dentistry, Oregon Health & Science University, School of Dentistry, Portland, Oregon, USA

JOSE AYUB, DDS
Visiting Scholar, Department of Preventive and Restorative Sciences, University of Pennsylvania School of Dental Medicine, Philadelphia, Pennsylvania, USA

ATAIS BACCHI, DDS, MS, PhD
Post-Graduate Program in Dentistry, Paulo Picanço School of Dentistry, Fortaleza, Ceará, Brazil

MARKUS B. BLATZ, DMD, PhD
Professor and Chair, Department of Preventive and Restorative Sciences, Assistant Dean for Digital Innovation and Professional Development, University of Pennsylvania School of Dental Medicine, Philadelphia, Pennsylvania, USA

DESPOINA BOMPOLAKI, DDS, MS
Associate Professor, Director of Clinical Restorative Dentistry, Oregon Health & Science University, Portland, Oregon, USA

ROBERTO RUGGIERO BRAGA, DDS, MS, PhD
Full Professor, Department of Biomaterials and Oral Biology, University of São Paulo, São Paulo, São Paulo, Brazil

MILENA CADENARO, DDS, MS, PhD
Full Professor, Department of Medical Sciences, University of Trieste, Trieste, Institute for Maternal and Child Health - IRCCS "Burlo Garofolo," Trieste, Italy

PAULO FRANCISCO CESAR, DDS, MS, PhD
Department of Biomaterials and Oral Biology, University of São Paulo – USP. Av Prof Lineu Prestes, São Paulo, São Paulo, Brazil

JULIAN CONEJO, DMD, MSc
Assistant Professor of Clinical Restorative Dentistry, Department of Preventive and Restorative Sciences, University of Pennsylvania School of Dental Medicine, Philadelphia, Pennsylvania, USA

YUEJIA DENG, BDS
Department of Biomedical Sciences, Texas A&M University College of Dentistry, Dallas, Texas, USA

CHRISTOPHER FELLOWS, DDS
Restorative Dentistry, Oregon Health & Science University, School of Dentistry, Portland, Oregon, USA

BRUNA MARIN FRONZA, DDS, MS, PhD
Post-doctoral Fellow, Department of Biomaterials and Oral Biology, University of São Paulo, São Paulo, São Paulo, Brazil

ANA PAULA FUGOLIN, DDS, MS, PhD
Assistant Professor, Restorative Dentistry, Oregon Health & Science University, Portland, Oregon, USA

YONGXI LIANG, BDS, PhD
Department of Biomedical Sciences, Texas A&M University College of Dentistry, Dallas, Texas, USA

XIAOHUA LIU, PhD
Professor, Department of Biomedical Sciences, Texas A&M University College of Dentistry, Dallas, Texas, USA

ERINNE BISSONNETTE LUBISICH, DMD
Assistant Professor, Director of Preclinical Restorative Dentistry, Oregon Health & Science University, Portland, Oregon, USA

IN-SUNG LUKE YEO, DDS, MS, PhD
Professor, Department of Prosthodontics, School of Dentistry and Dental Research Institute, Seoul National University, Jongro-Gu, Seoul, Korea

SPIRO J. MEGREMIS, PhD, MS
Director, Dental Materials and Devices Research, ADA Science & Research Institute (ADA SRI), LLC, Chicago, Illinois, USA

MARY ANNE S. MELO, DDS, MSc, PhD
Associate Professor, Program in Dental Biomedical Sciences, Division of Operative Dentistry, Department of General Dentistry, University of Maryland School of Dentistry, Baltimore, Maryland, USA

LAMIA MOKEEM, DDS, MS
Graduate Student, Program in Dental Biomedical Sciences, University of Maryland School of Dentistry, Baltimore, Maryland, USA

DAYANE OLIVEIRA, DDS, MS, PhD
Clinical Assistant Professor, Center for Dental Biomaterials, Department of Restorative and Dental Sciences, University of Florida College of Dentistry, Gainesville, Florida, USA

MATEUS GARCIA ROCHA, DDS, MS, PhD
Clinical Assistant Professor, Center for Dental Biomaterials, Department of Restorative and Dental Sciences, University of Florida College of Dentistry, Gainesville, Florida, USA

VINICIUS ROSA, DDS, MSc, PhD
Associate Professor, Director of Oral Care Health Innovations and Designs Singapore (ORCHIDS), Faculty of Dentistry, National University of Singapore, Singapore, Singapore

DIANA GABRIELA SOARES, DDS, MSc, PhD
Assistant Professor, Department of Operative Dentistry, Endodontics and Dental Materials, São Paulo University – USP, Bauru School of Dentistry, Bauru, São Paulo, Brazil

JIRUN SUN, MS, PhD
Senior Researcher, The Forsyth Institute, Harvard School of Dental Medicine Affiliate, Cambridge, Massachusetts, USA

HIDEHIKO WATANABE, DDS, MS
Restorative Dentistry, Oregon Health & Science University, School of Dentistry, Portland, Oregon, USA

Contents

The latest advancements in dentin bonding have focused on strategies to impair degradation mechanisms in order to extend the longevity of bonded interfaces. Protease inhibitors can reduce collagen degradation within the hybrid layer (HL). Collagen cross-linkers allow better adhesive infiltration and also inhibit proteases activity. Particles added to adhesive can promote mineral precipitation within the HL, reducing nanoleakage and micropermeability, besides possible antimicrobial and enzymatic inhibition effects. Most of these approaches are still experimental, and aspects of the adhesive under the clinician's control are still determinant for the long-term stability of adhesive restorations.

Continuous advancements in resin-based composites can make selection of the appropriate system a daunting task for the clinician. This review aims to simplify this process and clarify some new or controversial topics. Various types of composites for direct and indirect applications are discussed, including microfilled and microhybrid composites, nanocomposites, single shade, bulk fill, fiber-reinforced, high temperature/high pressure processed, CAD/CAM, and three-dimensional printable composites. Recent material advancements that lead to improved seal and toughness, degradation resistance, antimicrobial and self-healing capabilities are presented. Future directions are highlighted, such as the development of "smart" materials that are able to interact with the host environment.

This article focuses on the current understanding and concerns over the blue-light hazard when using dental light-curing units. It also provides information and safety protocols to guide the practitioner in making important decisions regarding dental personnel's health and the quality of dental restorations.

Bioactive materials for dental resin restorations are a rising field of investigation exploring treatment strategies for reducing the recurrence of carious lesions. The current effort has been directed toward developing dental materials that can inhibit biofilms and prevent tooth mineral loss. Bioactive resin materials have shown the potential to interfere with polymicrobial consortia in vivo and help maintain the lifespan of restorations.

Although the accuracy of direct digitization of oral structure has been improved, indirect digitization is still required in specific situations such as full-arch scanning. Once accurate images are imported, efficient designing can be achieved by CAD software. Although smile design using a 3-dimensional facial scan better predicts planned restorations, further improvement in virtual articulators is needed for complex cases. Computer-aided manufacturing can be offered in several formats such as chairside, laboratory, or centralized fabrications. The subtractive technique is mainly used for restorations, and many chairside CAM materials are available now, but the additive technique has the potential to save materials and an advantage in fabricating complex geometries. Limited evidence is available in applying CAD/CAM technologies in implant restorations. However, it is used to fabricate custom implant abutments and crowns from various materials such as titanium, zirconia, and PEEK and hybrid crowns using stock titanium base abutments.

The purpose of this study is to present current dental ceramic materials and processing methods. The clinical indication was emphasized on basis of the material's microstructure and composition. Studies of ceramic characterization were also discussed, as they impact the clinical indication and serve as a parameter for the development of new materials. The novel strategies were mostly found aiming to mimic the natural dental structures, provide mechanical reliability, and develop predictable restorations in terms of adaptation and design.

Resin-bonded ceramic restorations are common treatment options. Clinical longevity of resin-bonded ceramic restorations depends on the quality and durability of the resin-ceramic bond. The type and composition of the specific ceramic determines the selection of the most effective bonding protocol. Such protocol typically includes a surface pretreatment step followed by application of a priming agent. Understanding of fundamental ceramic properties and chemical compositions enables the clinician to make proper material selection decisions for clinically successful and long-lasting restorations. Based on research accrued over the past decades, this article reviews and discusses current resin-bonding protocols to most commonly used dental ceramics.

Surface characteristics are an important factor for long-term clinical success of dental implants. Alterations of implant surface characteristics accelerate or improve osseointegration by interacting with the physiology of bone healing. Dental implant surfaces have been traditionally modified at the microlevel. Recently, researchers have actively investigated nanomodifications in dental implants. This review explores implant surface modifications that enhance biological response at the interface between a bone and the implant.

Novel technologies and platforms have allowed significant breakthroughs in dental pulp tissue engineering. The development of injectable scaffolds that can be combined with stem cells, growth factors, or other bioactive compounds has enabled the regeneration of functional dental pulps able to secrete dentin in preclinical and clinical studies. Similarly, cell-homing technologies and scaffold-free strategies aim to modulate dental pulp self-regeneration mediated by resident stem cells and can evade some of the technical challenges related to cell-based tissue engineering strategies. This article will discuss emerging technologies and platforms for the clinical applications of dental pulp tissue engineering.

As a widespread chronical disease, periodontitis progressively destroys tooth-supporting structures (periodontium) and eventually leads to tooth loss. Therefore, regeneration of damaged/lost periodontal tissues has been a major subject in periodontal research. During periodontal tissue regeneration, biomaterials play pivotal roles in improving the outcome of the periodontal therapy. With the advancement of biomaterial science and engineering in recent years, new biomimetic materials and scaffolding fabrication technologies have been proposed for periodontal tissue regeneration. This article summarizes recent progress in periodontal tissue regeneration from a biomaterial perspective. First, various guide tissue regeneration/guide bone regeneration membranes and grafting biomaterials for periodontal tissue regeneration are overviewed. Next, the recent development of multifunctional scaffolding biomaterials for alveolar bone/periodontal ligament/cementum regeneration is summarized. Finally, clinical care points and perspectives on the use of biomimetic scaffolding materials to reconstruct the hierarchical periodontal tissues are provided.

The formal history of standards and dentistry in the United States goes back to World War I and was prompted by the government's need to buy large quantities of dental materials to treat "an army of teeth in disrepair." This article covers the use of scientific research to establish specifications and standards used to evaluate dental materials and products, and how a practitioner can use these standards to assure the safety and performance of the materials that they use in their everyday practice.

DENTAL CLINICS OF NORTH AMERICA

SERIES OF RELATED INTEREST

Atlas of the Oral and Maxillofacial Surgery Clinics

Oral and Maxillofacial Surgery Clinics

THE CLINICS ARE AVAILABLE ONLINE!
Access your subscription at:
www.theclinics.com

Preface

Advances in Biomaterials for Oral Health

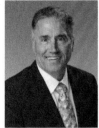 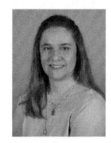 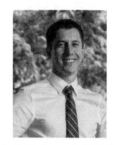

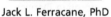

Jack L. Ferracane, PhD   Carmem S. Pfeifer, DDS, PhD   Luiz E. Bertassoni, DDS, PhD

Editors

The field of oral biomaterials continues to grow at a frantic pace, with the continual introduction of new products claiming important characteristics for improving oral health. Materials and technologies of extremely high quality are available to oral health care practitioners. In large part, the tremendous competition in the field essentially ensures that providers are supplied with excellent and appropriate tools to maintain the health of their patients. It is incumbent on these providers to be up-to-date with the latest developments, not only in terms of the various new products that have been introduced but also in terms of their ideal indications and the optimal ways for using them. It is for this reason that we have compiled this group of eleven outstanding articles from an internationally distinguished list of authors to provide an update and overview of oral biomaterials and technologies.

In the past, materials were developed for dentistry and oral health care with a primary focus on tissue replacement or augmentation, accompanied by minimal biological impact. The emphasis in many of the research and development initiatives today is on materials that are designed to interact with the biological environment to produce some beneficial effect, whether that be related to repairing or regenerating tissues or reducing or eliminating microbiological challenges. In addition, advances in digital imaging technology are greatly simplifying and facilitating many of the analog procedures used for many decades to create fixed and removable dental prostheses. Without a doubt, this is an exciting time to be an oral health care provider.

This issue is complete with articles addressing both traditional and new materials, but often looking at specific aspects related to their performance in the oral cavity and their interactions with biological tissues. For example, dental adhesives are addressed, but from the standpoint of how tooth surfaces may be modified to enhance bonding and make it more durable. These adhesives will be useful for the current and future generations of resin-based dental composites used in direct and indirect

Dent Clin N Am 66 (2022) xiii–xiv
https://doi.org/10.1016/j.cden.2022.05.001
0011-8532/22/© 2022 Published by Elsevier Inc.

restorations. Each of these resin-based materials is most frequently hardened with visible light-curing devices, but the professional must be aware of the potential blue light hazard when these devices are used. As discussed above, perhaps the new frontier in dental restoratives is "bioactive" materials, which is being designed for many different uses at this time. These materials have application in new restorative products, but also for modifying implant surfaces to minimize infection of the periodontium, as well as in active scaffolds for regenerating both periodontal and pulpal tissues. Advances in dental ceramics and the cements used to adhere them to teeth remain a critical and important mainstay of modern dentistry, as is the development of new technologies that facilitate the use of these materials. Finally, a look at the process by which standards are developed to assure the safety of dental products is presented.

This comprehensive set of articles will be helpful to clinical educators, practitioners, and researchers alike, who strive to have the most up-to-date information about the materials and systems available for providing optimal oral health care.

Jack L. Ferracane, PhD
Department of Restorative Dentistry
Oregon Health & Science University
2730 South Moody Avenue
Portland, OR 97201, USA

Carmem S. Pfeifer, DDS, PhD
Department of Restorative Dentistry
Oregon Health & Science University
2730 South Moody Avenue
Portland, OR 97201, USA

Luiz E. Bertassoni, DDS, PhD
Department of Restorative Dentistry
Oregon Health & Science University
2730 South Moody Avenue
Portland, OR 97201, USA

E-mail addresses:
ferracan@ohsu.edu (J.L. Ferracane)
pfeiferc@ohsu.edu (C.S. Pfeifer)
bertasso@ohsu.edu (L.E. Bertassoni)

Dental Adhesives—Surface Modifications of Dentin Structure for Stable Bonding

Bruna Marin Fronza, DDS, MS, PhD[a], Roberto Ruggiero Braga, DDS, MS, PhD[a,*],
Milena Cadenaro, DDS, MS, PhD[b,c]

KEYWORDS

- Dentin • Dentin bonding systems • Collagen • Matrix metalloproteinases
- Collagen cross-linking agents • MMP inhibitors • Bond strength • Zymography

KEY POINTS

- Resin hydrolysis and collagen degradation by endogenous enzymes influence the long-term integrity of bonded interfaces.
- Strategies to extend longevity of bonded interfaces include enzymatic inhibition, collagen cross-linking, and mineral precipitation within the hybrid layer.
- Proper and careful adhesive application by the dentist remains the foremost aspect to guarantee the longevity of bonded interfaces with currently available systems.

INTRODUCTION

Adhesive systems have been substantially improved over the years regarding their chemistry, interaction with dental substrates and with restorative materials, and clinical protocols.[1] Latest advancements have focused on reducing the number of steps and technique sensitivity, as well as on the development of strategies to extend the longevity of bonded interfaces. These included increasing the resistance of the resin components against hydrolysis and inhibiting enzymatic degradation of the collagen fibrils.[2–4]

Tjäderhane and colleagues (1998) first described the role of dentinal matrix metalloproteinases (MMPs), a group of endogenous peptidases, in the dentin matrix breakdown in caries lesions.[5] Pashley and colleagues (2004) then showed that the degradation of the collagen in acid-etched dentin is mediated by the activity of MMPs, activated during dentin bonding procedures[6] (**Fig. 1**). Besides MMPs, another

[a] Department of Biomaterials and Oral Biology, University of São Paulo, Av. Prof. Lineu Prestes, 2227, São Paulo, São Paulo 05508-000, Brazil; [b] Department of Medical Sciences, University of Trieste, Strada di Fiume 447, Trieste 34149, Italy; [c] Institute for Maternal and Child Health - IRCCS "Burlo Garofolo", Via dell'Istria 65/1, Trieste 34137, Italy
* Corresponding author. Av. Prof. Lineu Prestes, 2227, São Paulo, São Paulo 05508-000, Brazil.
E-mail address: rrbraga@usp.br

Dent Clin N Am 66 (2022) 503–515
https://doi.org/10.1016/j.cden.2022.05.002
0011-8532/22/© 2022 Elsevier Inc. All rights reserved.

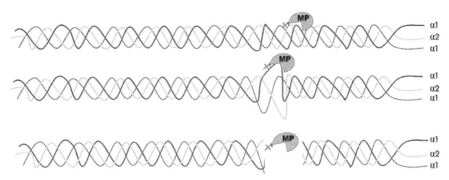

Fig. 1. Metalloproteinase (MP) breaks the collagen molecules, causing the loss of the triple helical conformation, resulting in fragments that will be slowly hydrolyzed by the proteolytic enzymes. (*Adapted from* de Moraes IQS, do Nascimento TG, da Silva AT, de Lira L, Parolia A, Porto I. Inhibition of matrix metalloproteinases: a troubleshooting for dentin adhesion. Restor Dent Endod. 2020;45(3):e31.)

class of enzymes has been identified in human dentin: cysteine proteases, which may contribute to the slow collagen degradation within the hybrid layer (HL) acting synergically with MMPs.[7] The elucidation of the role of endogenous proteases in the longevity of the HL prompted intense research activity aiming at inhibiting protease activity and/or increasing collagen resistance to enzymatic breakdown. This article describes the recent advances in dentin surface modification with the purpose of extending bond longevity.

PROTEASE INHIBITORS

Studies focused on MMPs inhibition in the last years show a great heterogeneity of molecules proposed: in a recent systematic review, 21 different inhibitors were identified.[8] Depending on the strategy chosen, the inhibitors can be used as an additional priming step after acid etching, included in primer formulations, or the adhesive resin.[9]

Chlorhexidine

A large portion of the literature on MMP inhibitors focuses on chlorhexidine (CHX), a common antimicrobial agent used in dentistry. The ability of CHX to inhibit the MMPs has been clearly demonstrated,[6] and since then, several studies have proven the efficacy of this biguanide compound in preserving the integrity and stability of the dentinal collagen in the HL and improving bond strength durability both in vivo and in vitro conditions.[10] CHX is readily available in clinical practice, and if applied at low concentrations (0.05%–0.2%) as an additional priming step on etched dentin, it effectively inhibits the enzymatic activity of MMPs[11] and improves the long-term bond strength.[12] Interestingly, it has been demonstrated that CHX can be retained within the HL even after 10 years of aging in vitro, maintaining its MMP-inhibitory properties.[11] Besides its use as a primer, CHX has also been added to adhesive formulations with encouraging results.[13]

The likely inhibitory mechanism of CHX against MMPs and cysteine cathepsins is linked to its ability to subtract zinc and calcium ions essential for the activity of these enzymes.[2,10] The cationic nature of CHX explains its ability to react with the anionic compounds of dentin contained in collagen but also in the inorganic matrix.[11]

Quaternary Ammonium Compounds

Similar to the CHX, other cationic molecules, such as quaternary ammonium compounds, may inhibit the collagenolytic activity of dentin endogenous enzymes. Benzalkonium chloride is a quaternary ammonium compound with antimicrobial and surfactant properties that has already been proved to be a MMPs inhibitor with an efficacy comparable to that of CHX, able to prolong the duration of the adhesive interface over time.[14,15] A quaternary ammonium methacrylate, 12-methacryloyloxydodecylpyridinium bromide (MDPB), integrated into a commercial adhesive system thanks to the presence of a resinous group, which has shown good ability to inhibit the MMPs activity.[16]

Therapeutic Drugs

Various therapeutic drugs used against different pathologic conditions have inhibiting properties on MMPs, and for this reason, their use in adhesive dentistry has been proposed. For instance, broad-spectrum antibiotics such as tetracycline and its analogs minocycline and doxycycline have cationic chelating properties and are capable of downregulation of MMPs mRNA expression, effectively blocking their activity.[2,10,17] The incorporation of nanotubes releasing doxycycline[18] and electrospun fibers containing doxycycline have been tested as fillers[19] in dental adhesives, leading to promising results in terms of MMPs inhibition. Nonetheless, the photo-oxidative stain of teeth caused by tetracyclines may impair the clinical use of these compounds in dentistry.[10]

Bisphosphonates are a class of drugs used in treating osteoporosis and Paget disease, which are effective inhibitors of MMPs produced by osteoclasts[17] by chelating zinc and calcium ions from the enzymes.[2] Their application in adhesive dentistry is promising,[20] even though the studies on bisphosphonates as MMP inhibitors in dentistry are still limited.

Other Inhibitors

Among the various molecules proposed, galardin is a specific synthetic MMP inhibitor effective against different MMPs at concentrations around 10 to 100 times lower than CHX.[2] When added to the primer of an E&R adhesive, galardin reduced the degradation of the HL after 1 year.[21]

Dimethyl sulfoxide (DMSO) has been recently proposed as a solvent in adhesive dentistry, being miscible in organic solvents, water and resin monomers commonly used in dentistry.[22] DMSO showed several beneficial properties for the adhesive interface, including a noteworthy inhibitory effect on MMPs when used as dentin pretreatment (**Box 1**).[23]

COLLAGEN CROSS-LINKING

Collagen strength and stiffness is related to its highly cross-linked structure. During the past 15 years, several synthetic and organic compounds capable of forming additional interfibrillar and intrafibrillar cross-links have been tested as a strategy to improve the longevity of the adhesive/dentin interface (**Box 2**). Although earlier investigations proposed long application times to effect maintenance of interfacial integrity,[24] cross-linkers soon started to be tested in clinically feasible protocols, for instance as an extra priming step after phosphoric acid etching or the application of the self-etching primer,[25] mixed to universal adhesive systems,[26] or mixed to phosphoric acid.[27]

How Do Collagen Cross-Linkers Contribute to Dentin Bond Stability?

The success of adhesive restorations, both in the short-term and long-term, relies on the effective adhesive infiltration within the collagen network. In that sense,

Box 1
Substances tested as protease inhibitors

Group	Inhibitor
Cationic compounds	• 0.2%–2% CHX gluconate
	• Quaternary ammonium compounds (MDPB)
Antibiotics	• Minocycline
	• Doxycycline
Bisphosphonates	• Polyvinylphosphonic acid
Other inhibitors	• Galardin
	• SB-3CT 2-[[(4-Phenoxyphenyl)sulfonyl]methyl]thiirane
	• E-64 L-trans-Epoxysuccinyl-leucylamido(4-guanidino)butane
	• Odanacatib
	• DMSO

cross-linking was shown to increase the stiffness of the collagen fibrils,[28] preventing their collapse when dried[29] and allowing for better resin infiltration. The superior quality of HLs obtained in dentin samples pretreated with different cross-linkers explains the higher initial bond strength values in comparison to nontreated dentin substrates.[30,31] Yet, the real benefits of collagen cross-linkers are observed after prolonged storage. Several in vitro studies testing different cross-linkers attested to the stability of the bonded interface after 1 to 5 years.[32,33] In part, this effect can be ascribed to better resin infiltration because poorly infiltrated demineralized collagen networks are more susceptible to endogenous proteases. Moreover, because voids in the HL are filled with dentinal fluid, suboptimal adhesive infiltration increases the hydrolysis of the resin component.[10]

Notwithstanding, to a large extent preservation of the bonded interfaces is explained by the inhibitory effect of cross-linkers over protease activity. The proposed inhibition mechanisms include (1) irreversible changes in their tertiary structure by the establishment of multiple cross-links in their catalytic sites, (2) alosteric control, that is, the modification of noncatalytic domains also involved in protease activity, and (3) indirectly, by cross-linking functional domains of noncollagen proteins present in dentin involved in MMP activity (eg, dentin matrix protein-1/DMP-1 and bone sialoprotein/BSP).[34] Protease inhibition by cross-linkers is a long-term effect, as demineralized dentin beams treated with cross-linkers showed less protease activity than the untreated control after 6 months.[35] In situ zymography, used to quantify MMP activity in bonded interfaces, showed lower protease activity in interfaces treated with cross-linkers after 1[30,36] and 5 years[37] (**Fig. 2**).

Box 2
Substances tested as collagen cross-linkers

Source	Group	Examples
Synthetic	Aldehydes	GA, acrolein
	Carbodiimides	EDC, DCC
Natural	Riboflavins	RF, riboflavin-5-phosphate
	Proanthocyanidins	GSE, GTE, CJE

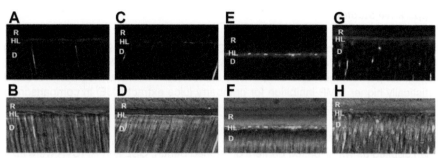

Fig. 2. Representative examples of in-situ zymography of the resin–dentin interfaces after 1 year in artificial saliva. Green fluorescence indicates protease activity. Dentin treated with a universal adhesive in self-etching (SE) mode (*A, B*); universal adhesive (SE) + 0.5 M carbodiimide, applied for 1 min between the application of 2 layers of the adhesive (*C, D*); universal adhesive in etch-and-rinse (ER) mode (*E, F*); and universal adhesive (ER)+ 0.5 M carbodiimide for 1 minute, after acid etching (*G, H*). D, dentin; HL, hybrid layer; R, resin composite. (*From* Comba A, Maravić T, Villalta V, et al. Effect of an ethanol cross-linker on universal adhesive. Dental Materials. 2020;36(12):1645-1654.)

Cross-Linkers

The characteristics of the main compounds tested as collagen cross-linkers are described below.

Glutaraldehyde

This is an aliphatic molecule containing 5 carbon atoms and one aldehyde (−COH) group in each extremity, capable of establishing chemical bonds with collagen amino (−NH$_2$) groups, forming intramolecular and intermolecular cross-links.[28] Unfortunately, glutaraldehyde (GA) is cytotoxic, which prevents its clinical use.[38]

Carbodiimides

N,N'-dicyclohexylcarbodiimide (DCC) and 1-ethyl-3-(3-dimethylaminopropyl)carbodiimide (EDC) (see **Box 2**) have a basic structure represented as R_1-N=C=N-R_2 (where R_1 and R_2 can be, for instance, a methyl group and an amino group). They are considered "zero-length" cross-linkers, which mediate the formation of an amide cross-link between collagen carboxyl and amine groups, without adding extra groups in between.[39]

Riboflavin

Riboflavin (RF) is a water-soluble, nontoxic photosensitizer capable of releasing oxygen-reactive species when exposed to ultraviolet A (UVA) light (368 nm) and induce the formation of new cross-links.[40] Blue light (470–480 nm) can also be used but it is less efficient than UVA.[41]

Proanthocyanidines

These belong to a group of naturally occurring plant metabolite bioflavonoids with complex molecular structures containing one aliphatic and multiple phenolic hydroxyl groups.[24,42] The cross-linking mechanisms promoted by proanthocyanidines (PACs) include hydrogen bonding and hydrophobic interactions with proline groups of the collagen at intrafibrillar and interfibrillar levels.[43] Collagen cross-linking with PACs leads to dehydration of the fibrils, improving its resistance to collagenases.[44]

Comparative Studies

Proteolytic activity

Cross-linkers were shown to reduce MMP-2, MMP-8, and MMP-9 activities by 21% to 70% after treatment times of 1 or 5 minutes, with grape seed extract (GSE) showing the highest percentages, and GA and RF, the lowest.[45] In situ zymography revealed statistically higher MMP inhibition for cranberry juice extract (CJE) in comparison to green tea extract (GTE) and GSE.[39]

Long-term stability of bonded interfaces

When applied as water-based primers on etched dentin, GSE and RF/UVA were able to maintain bond strength values of etch-and-rinse, 2-step adhesives to dentin during an 18-month period. When GA was used as primer, however, bond strength was stable only with one of the tested adhesives.[38] Indentation fracture toughness (iFT) test was used to assess the efficacy of water-based primers containing GSE, RF/UVA, or GA associated with universal adhesives. After 6-month storage in artificial saliva, only the specimens treated with GSE showed higher iFT in relation to the control.[25] Acid-eroded dentin samples treated with water-based primers containing GSE or RF/blue light following phosphoric acid etching showed stable microtensile bond strength values after 2-year storage in water.[32]

Is the Use of Collagen Cross-Linkers Clinically Viable?

Dentin biomodification using collagen cross-linkers seems to be a promising strategy to extend the durability of bonded interfaces. However, their application as primers would significantly increase chair-side time. In order to avoid adding an additional step to the bonding procedure, attempts have been made of adding cross-linkers to the adhesive or to the etchant.

Etchants

Proanthocianidins remain effective at lower pH and, therefore, can be mixed with phosphoric acid. Bonded interfaces obtained with the use of an experimental etchant containing 2% GSE, 20% ethanol, and 10% phosphoric acid associated with 2-step, etch-and-rinse commercial adhesive showed no reduction in bond strength after 6 months[46] and 1 year of storage,[31] as opposed to specimens where dentin was conditioned with 35% phosphoric acid. The same etchant formulation was shown to increase the immediate bond strength to caries-affected dentin by nearly 70% and significantly reduced MMP activity not only in relation to the control group (37% phosphoric acid) but also to specimens treated with CHX.[27] However, the incorporation of GSE to 37% phosphoric acid resulted in lower bond strength values in relation to the control etchant, even though the increase in cross-linking was verified by infrared spectroscopy.[47]

Adhesive systems

RF added to commercial universal adhesives resulted in less severe reductions in bond strength after 6 months of storage in artificial saliva in relation to the respective controls without the cross-linker.[26] A clinical study evaluated the effect of adding GSE to a commercial 2-step, etch-and-rinse adhesive system. After 2 years, the retention rates of restorations of noncarious cervical lesions placed with the modified adhesives were statistically lower than that of the control adhesive. Authors attributed the results to reduced degree of conversion of the adhesives, as proanthocyanidins are free-radicals scavengers.[48]

THE USE OF PARTICLES IN ADHESIVES

Several *in vitro* studies have demonstrated the beneficial effects of the addition of ion-releasing particles in experimental and commercial adhesives as a strategy to reduce adhesive degradation (**Box 3**).[3,9,49]

Silver ions can induce bacteria cell lysis, prevent bacterial DNA replication, and disrupt bacterial protein synthesis.[50] Adhesives containing silver-based particles present antibiofilm properties and lower risk for secondary caries development.[51,52] Other ions such as fluoride, zinc, and copper have been identified as MMPs inhibitors because they can bind to their specific sites and induce conformational changes that hinder enzyme activity.[53] Zinc ions can also bind to specific sites on the exposed collagen fibrils and modify their spatial configuration, protecting sensitive cleavage sites from the MMPs.[54] The addition of ZnO particles to a commercial etch-and-rinse, 2-step adhesive was shown to reduce collagen degradation after 4 weeks.[55]

Calcium-releasing particles, such as amorphous calcium phosphate (ACP), α-tricalcium phosphate, β-tricalcium phosphate (β-TCP), dicalcium phosphate dihydrate, octacalcium phosphate, and hydroxyapatite, have been tested as additives in experimental adhesives to promote mineral precipitation and replace water from poorly resin-infiltrated spaces within the HL.[56–60] Mineral precipitates may also reduce enzymatic activity by electrostatic interactions with some MMPs. Calcium-releasing particles can be also doped with metallic oxides as a strategy to increase the MMP inhibitory effect.[3]

Remineralization of the HL not only increases the mechanical properties of the interphase but was also shown to reduce hydrolytic degradation and to inhibit protease activity.[61] Bioactive glasses (BAGs) and calcium silicates (CaSi) release calcium ions that, along with phosphate ions present in physiologic fluids, promote mineral deposition. CaSi also releases hydroxyl ions from its crystalline calcium hydroxide phase, which increases local pH and favors mineral precipitation, antimicrobial action, and MMP inhibition.[62] Mineral precipitation (**Fig. 3**) within the HL reduced the micropermeability of dentin–resin interfaces for adhesives containing 30% to 40% of BAGs or CaSi fillers after 3 to 6 months storage in phosphate-containing medium, in comparison to unfilled adhesives.[56,57,62,63] The elastic modulus of the HL increased after 3 months for adhesives loaded with 40 wt% BAG or 33 wt% CaSi and β-TCP, whereas this property was reduced when particles were absent.[57,63] The application

Box 3	
Particles and their effects on bonded interfaces	
Particle	**Observed Effects**
Silver nanoparticles	Antimicrobial activity
Metallic oxides	Inhibition of enzymatic activity and reduced collagen degradation, antimicrobial activity, mineral deposition, higher long-term bond strength
BAGs	Reduction of micropermeability and nanoleakage of the HL, higher long-term bond strength, and remineralization of caries-affected dentin
CaSi	Mineral deposition, enhancement of HL mechanical properties, bond strength preservation, micropermeability and nanoleakage reduction
Calcium orthophosphates	Mineral precipitation, nanoleakage reduction, and improvement in bond strength

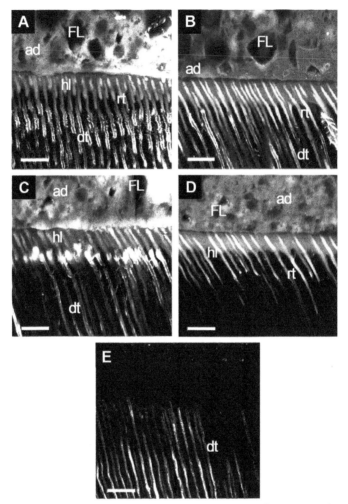

Fig. 3. Resin–dentin interfaces of experimental etch-and-rinse adhesive doped with calcium silicate-based microfillers immersed in simulated body fluid (SBF) solution for 24 hours or 6 months. Orange fluorescence is a calcium-chelator dye. Images indicate the remineraliza-tion of areas previously detected as poor-resin infiltrated zones of the resin–dentin inter-face. (*A*) Resin–dentin interface created with sodium–calcium–aluminum–magnesium silicate hydroxide fillers, where mineral deposition is identified within the adhesive layer (ad), the HL, and along the walls of dentinal tubules (dt), besides the fillers inside the resin tags (rt). (*B*) Resin–dentin interface created with aluminum–magnesium–carbonate hydrox-ide hydrates fillers showing Ca-deposits within the ad, HL, walls of the dt and rt after 6 months of SBF immersion. (*C*) Resin–dentin interface created with titanium oxide fillers demonstrate intense calcium deposition at bottom of HL, besides Ca-mineral within ad, HL, and dt. (*D*) Resin–dentin interface also with titanium oxide but after 6 months, showing Ca-mineral presence at the bottom and within the HL, dt, and rt. (*E*) Resin–dentin interface created with no-fillers adhesive (control) in which it is possible to note the absence of cal-cium deposition both within the HL and ad. Only the walls of the dentinal dt were stained by the fluorescent dye. (*From* Profeta AC, Mannocci F, Foxton R, et al. Experimental etch-and-rinse adhesives doped with bioactive calcium silicate-based micro-fillers to generate therapeutic resin-dentin interfaces. *Dent Mater.* 2013;29(7):729-741.)

of BAG particles to dentin as pretreatment primers in combination with a commercial adhesive also resulted in higher elastic modulus values of the HL.[64]

The association of ion-releasing particles with biomimetic analogs of noncollagenous proteins such as poli(acrylic) and poly(aspartic) acids has been suggested.[3] These molecules act as stabilizers and templates to guide apatite growth in an oriented manner along within collagen matrix. Dental adhesives containing ion-releasing fillers treated with polyacrylic acid have been shown to regulate apatite precipitation.[56] Polyaspartic acid in combination with Si-ACP nanoparticles added into self-etch adhesives promoted the remineralization of the bottom of the HL after 3 months.[60]

Studies on long-term dentin bond strength involving particle-containing adhesives have shown inconsistent results. Some studies report no loss in microtensile bond strength, whereas adhesion values are significantly decreased for control unfilled groups.[55,62,64] However, no difference between adhesives with or without particles was found in other studies.[56,57] Indeed, particles size and concentration are determinants for the mechanical behavior and bond strength of adhesives.[59,65] Besides, the lack of a strong chemical interaction between the resin matrix and of the particles jeopardizes stress distribution and can significantly reduce the material's mechanical properties.[59,66]

Two clinical studies evaluated the use of particles in adhesive systems. The addition of 0.1 wt% copper nanoparticles in a commercial one-bottle universal adhesive applied in etch-and-rinse mode improved the retention rate and marginal sealing of noncarious cervical lesions restorations after 18 months. These findings were attributed to copper protective action against collagen degradation.[67] However, the use of biosilicate particles (BAG) in different classes of adhesives did not improve the clinical performance of posterior restorations after 18 months.[68]

FINAL REMARKS

Adhesive systems have been substantially improved over the years regarding their chemistry, interaction with dental substrates and restorative materials, and technique sensitivity. Notwithstanding, the longevity of bonded interfaces remains a clinical concern. The strategies described here to reduce collagen degradation represent pathways to increase the long-term success of adhesive procedures. However, clinical studies are necessary to confirm some of the promising results obtained in vitro.

CLINICS CARE POINTS

- Most of the strategies to improve the durability of the adhesive interface are still experimental and need further investigations to be transferred to the clinical practice.
- CHX applied in low concentrations (0.05–0.2%) as an additional priming step on etched dentin to inhibit the MMPs is the only protocol that can be easily applied in clinical practice.
- The dentist should be aware that careful placement of the adhesive system is the first step to guarantee a stable bonding.

DISCLOSURE

The authors have nothing to disclose.

REFERENCES

1. Van Meerbeek B, Yoshihara K, Van Landuyt K, et al. From Buonocore's Pioneering Acid-Etch Technique to Self-Adhering Restoratives. A Status

Perspective of Rapidly Advancing Dental Adhesive Technology. J Adhes Dent 2020;22(1):7–34.

2. Frassetto A, Breschi L, Turco G, et al. Mechanisms of degradation of the hybrid layer in adhesive dentistry and therapeutic agents to improve bond durability–A literature review. Dent Mater 2016;32(2):e41–53.

3. Braga RR, Fronza BM. The use of bioactive particles and biomimetic analogues for increasing the longevity of resin-dentin interfaces: A literature review. Dent Mater J 2020;39(1):62–8.

4. Perdigão J. Current perspectives on dental adhesion: (1) Dentin adhesion - not there yet. Jpn Dent Sci Rev 2020;56(1):190–207.

5. Tjäderhane L, Larjava H, Sorsa T, et al. The activation and function of host matrix metalloproteinases in dentin matrix breakdown in caries lesions. J Dent Res 1998; 77(8):1622–9.

6. Pashley DH, Tay FR, Yiu C, et al. Collagen degradation by host-derived enzymes during aging. J Dent Res 2004;83(3):216–21.

7. Mazzoni A, Tjäderhane L, Checchi V, et al. Role of dentin MMPs in caries progression and bond stability. J Dent Res 2015;94(2):241–51.

8. Kiuru O, Sinervo J, Vähänikkilä H, et al. MMP Inhibitors and Dentin Bonding: Systematic Review and Meta-Analysis. Int J Dent 2021;2021:9949699.

9. Münchow EA, Bottino MC. Recent Advances in Adhesive Bonding - The Role of Biomolecules, Nanocompounds, and Bonding Strategies in Enhancing Resin Bonding to Dental Substrates. Curr Oral Health Rep 2017;4(3):215–27.

10. Breschi L, Maravic T, Cunha SR, et al. Dentin bonding systems: From dentin collagen structure to bond preservation and clinical applications. Dent Mater 2018;34(1):78–96.

11. Breschi L, Maravic T, Comba A, et al. Chlorhexidine preserves the hybrid layer in vitro after 10-years aging. Dent Mater 2020;36(5):672–80.

12. Zhang X, Wang L, Liu S, et al. Evaluation of the bond strength of chlorhexidine incorporated into the adhesive system composition: A PRISMA guided meta-analysis. J Dent Sci 2020;15(3):315–28.

13. da Silva EM, de Sá Rodrigues CU, de Oliveira Matos MP, et al. Experimental etch-and-rinse adhesive systems containing MMP-inhibitors: Physicochemical characterization and resin-dentin bonding stability. J Dent 2015;43(12):1491–7.

14. Sabatini C, Scheffel DL, Scheffel RH, et al. Inhibition of endogenous human dentin MMPs by Gluma. Dent Mater 2014;30(7):752–8.

15. Comba A, Maravic T, Valente L, et al. Effect of benzalkonium chloride on dentin bond strength and endogenous enzymatic activity. J Dent 2019;85:25–32.

16. Tezvergil-Mutluay A, Agee KA, Mazzoni A, et al. Can quaternary ammonium methacrylates inhibit matrix MMPs and cathepsins? Dent Mater 2015;31(2): e25–32.

17. Boelen GJ, Boute L, d'Hoop J, et al. Matrix metalloproteinases and inhibitors in dentistry. Clin Oral Investig 2019;23(7):2823–35.

18. Palasuk J, Windsor LJ, Platt JA, et al. Doxycycline-loaded nanotube-modified adhesives inhibit MMP in a dose-dependent fashion. Clin Oral Investig 2018;22(3): 1243–52.

19. Münchow EA, da Silva AF, Piva E, et al. Development of an antibacterial and anti-metalloproteinase dental adhesive for long-lasting resin composite restorations. J Mater Chem B 2020;8(47):10797–811.

20. Tezvergil-Mutluay A, Agee KA, Hoshika T, et al. The inhibitory effect of polyvinylphosphonic acid on functional matrix metalloproteinase activities in human demineralized dentin. Acta Biomater 2010;6(10):4136–42.

21. Breschi L, Martin P, Mazzoni A, et al. Use of a specific MMP-inhibitor (galardin) for preservation of hybrid layer. Dent Mater 2010;26(6):571–8.

22. Stape THS, Tjäderhane L, Abuna G, et al. Optimization of the etch-and-rinse technique: New perspectives to improve resin-dentin bonding and hybrid layer integrity by reducing residual water using dimethyl sulfoxide pretreatments. Dent Mater 2018;34(7):967–77.

23. Stape THS, Mutluay MM, Tjäderhane L, et al. The pursuit of resin-dentin bond durability: Simultaneous enhancement of collagen structure and polymer network formation in hybrid layers. Dent Mater 2021;37(7):1083–95.

24. Bedran-Russo AK, Pereira PN, Duarte WR, et al. Application of crosslinkers to dentin collagen enhances the ultimate tensile strength. J Biomed Mater Res B Appl Biomater 2007;80(1):268–72.

25. Parise Gré C, Pedrollo Lise D, Ayres AP, et al. Do collagen cross-linkers improve dentin's bonding receptiveness? Dent Mater 2018;34(11):1679–89.

26. Fu C, Deng S, Koneski I, et al. Multiscale in-vitro analysis of photo-activated riboflavin incorporated in an experimental universal adhesive. J Mech Behav Biomed Mater 2020;112:104082.

27. Hass V, da Maceno Oliveira TB, Cardenas AFM, et al. Is it possible for a simultaneous biomodification during acid etching on naturally caries-affected dentin bonding? Clin Oral Investig 2021;25(6):3543–53.

28. Bedran-Russo AK, Pashley DH, Agee K, et al. Changes in stiffness of demineralized dentin following application of collagen crosslinkers. J Biomed Mater Res B Appl Biomater 2008;86(2):330–4.

29. Liu R, Fang M, Xiao Y, et al. The effect of transient proanthocyanidins preconditioning on the cross-linking and mechanical properties of demineralized dentin. J Mater Sci Mater Med 2011;22(11):2403–11.

30. Comba A, Maravić T, Villalta V, et al. Effect of an ethanol cross-linker on universal adhesive. Dental Mater 2020;36(12):1645–54.

31. Loguercio AD, Malaquias P, Dos Santos FP, et al. Acid Etching with Modified Phosphoric Acid to Increase the Longevity of the Bonded Interface. J Adhes Dent 2017;195–201.

32. de Siqueira FSF, Hilgemberg B, Araujo LCR, et al. Improving bonding to eroded dentin by using collagen cross-linking agents: 2 years of water storage. Clin Oral Investig 2020;24(2):809–22.

33. Mazzoni A, Angeloni V, Comba A, et al. Cross-linking effect on dentin bond strength and MMPs activity. Dent Mater 2018;34(2):288–95.

34. Liu Y, Tjaderhane L, Breschi L, et al. Limitations in bonding to dentin and experimental strategies to prevent bond degradation. J Dent Res 2011;90(8):953–68.

35. Seseogullari-Dirihan R, Mutluay MM, Pashley DH, et al. Is the inactivation of dentin proteases by crosslinkers reversible? Dent Mater 2017;33(2):e62–8.

36. Mazzoni A, Angeloni V, Sartori N, et al. Substantivity of Carbodiimide Inhibition on Dentinal Enzyme Activity over Time. J Dent Res 2017;96(8):902–8.

37. Maravic T, Mancuso E, Comba A, et al. Dentin Cross-linking Effect of Carbodiimide After 5 Years. J Dent Res 2021;100(10):1090–8.

38. Hass V, Luque-Martinez IV, Gutierrez MF, et al. Collagen cross-linkers on dentin bonding: Stability of the adhesive interfaces, degree of conversion of the adhesive, cytotoxicity and in situ MMP inhibition. Dent Mater 2016;32(6):732–41.

39. Wang Y, Green A, Yao X, et al. Cranberry juice extract rapidly protects demineralized dentin against digestion and inhibits its gelatinolytic activity. Materials (Basel) 2021;14(13):3637.

40. Spoerl E, Huhle M, Seiler T. Induction of Cross-links in Corneal Tissue. Exp Eye Res 1998;66(1):97–103.
41. Fawzy AS, Nitisusanta LI, Iqbal K, et al. Riboflavin as a dentin crosslinking agent: ultraviolet A versus blue light. Dent Mater 2012;28(12):1284–91.
42. Reis M, Zhou B, Alania Y, et al. Unveiling structure-activity relationships of proanthocyanidins with dentin collagen. Dent Mater 2021;37(11):1633–44.
43. Vidal CMP, Leme AA, Aguiar TR, et al. Mimicking the Hierarchical Functions of Dentin Collagen Cross-Links with Plant Derived Phenols and Phenolic Acids. Langmuir 2014;30(49):14887–93.
44. Liu Y, Chen M, Yao X, et al. Enhancement in dentin collagen's biological stability after proanthocyanidins treatment in clinically relevant time periods. Dental Mater 2013;29(4):485–92.
45. Seseogullari-Dirihan R, Apollonio F, Mazzoni A, et al. Use of crosslinkers to inactivate dentin MMPs. Dent Mater 2016;32(3):423–32.
46. Hass V, Luque-Martinez I, Muñoz MA, et al. The effect of proanthocyanidin-containing 10% phosphoric acid on bonding properties and MMP inhibition. Dent Mater 2016;32(3):468–75.
47. De-Paula DM, Lomonaco D, Ponte AMP, et al. Influence of collagen cross-linkers addition in phosphoric acid on dentin biomodification and bonding of an etch-and-rinse adhesive. Dent Mater 2020;36(1):e1–8.
48. de Souza LC, Rodrigues NS, Cunha DA, et al. Two-year clinical evaluation of proanthocyanidins added to a two-step etch-and-rinse adhesive. J Dent 2019; 81:7–16.
49. Farooq I, Ali S, Al-Saleh S, et al. Synergistic Effect of Bioactive Inorganic Fillers in Enhancing Properties of Dentin Adhesives-A Review. Polymers (Basel) 2021; 13(13):2169.
50. Noronha VT, Paula AJ, Duran G, et al. Silver nanoparticles in dentistry. Dent Mater 2017;33(10):1110–26.
51. Kramer N, Mohwald M, Lucker S, et al. Effect of microparticulate silver addition in dental adhesives on secondary caries in vitro. Clin Oral Investig 2015;19(7): 1673–81.
52. Dutra-Correa M, Leite A, de Cara S, et al. Antibacterial effects and cytotoxicity of an adhesive containing low concentration of silver nanoparticles. J Dent 2018;77: 66–71.
53. de Souza AP, Gerlach RF, Line SR. Inhibition of human gingival gelatinases (MMP-2 and MMP-9) by metal salts. Dent Mater 2000;16(2):103–8.
54. Osorio R, Yamauti M, Osorio E, et al. Zinc-doped dentin adhesive for collagen protection at the hybrid layer. Eur J Oral Sci 2011;119(5):401–10.
55. Toledano M, Yamauti M, Ruiz-Requena ME, et al. A ZnO-doped adhesive reduced collagen degradation favouring dentine remineralization. J Dent 2012; 40(9):756–65.
56. Wang Z, Shen Y, Haapasalo M, et al. Polycarboxylated microfillers incorporated into light-curable resin-based dental adhesives evoke remineralization at the mineral-depleted dentin. J Biomater Sci Polym Ed 2014;25(7):679–97.
57. Sauro S, Osorio R, Osorio E, et al. Novel light-curable materials containing experimental bioactive micro-fillers remineralise mineral-depleted bonded-dentine interfaces. J Biomater Sci Polym Ed 2013;24(8):940–56.
58. Garcia IM, Leitune VCB, Samuel SMW, et al. Influence of Different Calcium Phosphates on an Experimental Adhesive Resin. J Adhes Dent 2017;19(5):379–84.
59. Al-Hamdan RS, Almutairi B, Kattan HF, et al. Influence of Hydroxyapatite Nanospheres in Dentin Adhesive on the Dentin Bond Integrity and Degree of

Conversion: A Scanning Electron Microscopy (SEM), Raman, Fourier Transform-Infrared (FTIR), and Microtensile Study. Polymers (Basel) 2020;12(12):2948.

60. Wu Z, Wang X, Wang Z, et al. Self-Etch Adhesive as a Carrier for ACP Nanoprecursors to Deliver Biomimetic Remineralization. ACS Appl Mater Inter 2017;9(21): 17710–7.

61. Gu LS, Huffman BP, Arola DD, et al. Changes in stiffness of resin-infiltrated demineralized dentin after remineralization by a bottom-up biomimetic approach. Acta Biomater 2010;6(4):1453–61.

62. Profeta AC, Mannocci F, Foxton R, et al. Experimental etch-and-rinse adhesives doped with bioactive calcium silicate-based micro-fillers to generate therapeutic resin-dentin interfaces. Dent Mater 2013;29(7):729–41.

63. Sauro S, Osorio R, Watson TF, et al. Therapeutic effects of novel resin bonding systems containing bioactive glasses on mineral-depleted areas within the bonded-dentine interface. J Mater Sci Mater Med 2012;23(6):1521–32.

64. Bauer J, Silva ESA, Carvalho EM, et al. Dentin pretreatment with 45S5 and niobophosphate bioactive glass: Effects on pH, antibacterial, mechanical properties of the interface and microtensile bond strength. J Mech Behav Biomed Mater 2019; 90:374–80.

65. Belli R, Kreppel S, Petschelt A, et al. Strengthening of dental adhesives via particle reinforcement. J Mech Behav Biomed Mater 2014;37:100–8.

66. Balbinot GS, Collares FM, Herpich TL, et al. Niobium containing bioactive glasses as remineralizing filler for adhesive resins. Dent Mater 2020;36(2):221–8.

67. Matos TP, Gutierrez MF, Hanzen TA, et al. 18-month clinical evaluation of a copper-containing universal adhesive in non-carious cervical lesions: A double-blind, randomized controlled trial. J Dent 2019;90:103219.

68. Pintado-Palomino K, de Almeida C, da Motta RJG, et al. Clinical, double blind, randomized controlled trial of experimental adhesive protocols in caries-affected dentin. Clin Oral Investig 2019;23(4):1855–64.

Resin-Based Composites for Direct and Indirect Restorations

Clinical Applications, Recent Advances, and Future Trends

Despoina Bompolaki, DDS, MS*, Erinne Bissonnette Lubisich, DMD,
Ana Paula Fugolin, DDS, MS, PhD

KEYWORDS

- Composite resin • Microhybrid composites • Nanocomposites
- CAD/CAM composites • Indirect composites • Degradation • Antibacterial
- Self-healing

KEY POINTS

- Both microhybrid and nanohybrid/nanofilled composites provide esthetic appearance and high strength, making them an acceptable material option for the most clinical situations requiring a direct esthetic restoration.
- Although single-shade composites can simplify shade-matching procedures, their capabilities may be more limited in challenging esthetic scenarios, such as when needing to mask a dark substructure.
- High-temperature/high-pressure polymerization of resin-based composites leads to increased mechanical properties and reduction of polymerization shrinkage. These materials can be used in a variety of indirect applications, including posterior partial coverage restorations, crowns, and veneers, with acceptable short-term and medium-term clinical outcomes.
- Composite resins with antibacterial properties can decrease biofilm formation and acid production, preventing the development of secondary caries. Self-healing composites aim to impede crack propagation and repair any damage that may occur within the material.
- Future resin-based restorative dental materials might be capable of a dynamic interaction with the host environment, using uniquely coded instructions embedded in their chemical structure that enable them to perform a desired function on demand.

Restorative Dentistry, Oregon Health & Science University, 2730 S Moody Ave, Room 10N070, Portland, OR 97201, USA
* Corresponding author.
E-mail address: bompolak@ohsu.edu

Dent Clin N Am 66 (2022) 517–536
https://doi.org/10.1016/j.cden.2022.05.003
0011-8532/22/© 2022 Elsevier Inc. All rights reserved.

INTRODUCTION

During the last 70 years, resin composite materials have transformed restorative dentistry[1] and have become the most frequently used direct restorative material,[2] allowing dental practitioners to provide cost-effective, esthetic restorations.[1,3] For the most part, current dental composites possess adequate mechanical properties for use in all areas of the mouth,[4] although care must still be taken when placing these restorations in high load-bearing areas.[4] Selection of the appropriate composite system is critical to the success of the restoration[5] because resin composites are available in a variety of formulations and each has its own strengths and weaknesses.

At the same time, the increased use of resin-based composites has led to deeper understanding of their clinical limitations and shortcomings. Polymerization shrinkage, gap formation, bacterial leakage, secondary caries, crack propagation, and fracture[6] are still associated with the use of composite resins and pose a challenge to dental practitioners, who spend a significant portion of their time replacing composite restorations. This well-established knowledge of the material's long-term clinical behavior has been the guiding force toward some recent groundbreaking laboratory advancements, including the development of self-healed and antimicrobial composites.[7–11]

Given the ever-expanding use of composite resins and the development of new materials that are expected to be introduced in dental market in the near future, there is a critical need not only for a foundational understanding of the different types of resin composites but also for establishing clinical guidelines that will aid the practitioner during material selection for each individual case.

RESIN-BASED COMPOSITES FOR DIRECT RESTORATIONS

Resin composites for direct intraoral application generally consist of 4 components: organic matrix, inorganic filler particles, initiator system, and coupling agent.[12] Inorganic filler evolution has primarily involved the progressive manipulation of the particle size and distribution to enhance material properties. Appropriately, direct resin composites are often categorized based on the size of the filler particle. Macrofill composites, introduced in the 1970s, exhibited significant wear and poor esthetic properties. They were replaced with microfill composites, which have good esthetic properties and are highly polishable but have poor mechanical properties due to the very small particle size that impedes sufficient filler loading.[4] Historically, advancements in resin composites have led to either an increase in strength or an increase in esthetics, but not an increase in both,[12] until the introduction of current minifill/microhybrid composites, which can be used in virtually every clinical situation with acceptable results.[4,12] The most recent progress in filler size was introduced with the nanocomposites, which optimize both esthetic and mechanical properties[12] (**Table 1**). **Table 2** summarizes the clinical indications for each different type of composite.

Resin-Based Composites for Anterior Direct Restorations

Modern composite resins allow the clinician to create a restoration that blends well with the surrounding tooth structure, leading to superior esthetic results.[13] Esthetics are of utmost importance in anterior restorations, necessitating precise color matching and polishing ability,[14] which further enhances esthetic outcomes via interaction with incident light. Two systematic reviews on the clinical performance of direct anterior composite restorations identified restoration fracture and marginal degradation as the most frequent reasons for definitive failure of restorations, with color mismatch and marginal discoloration identified as most common reasons for relative failures, nevertheless leading to replacement.[15,16]

Table 1
Overview of composite types, characteristics, and clinical considerations

Composite Type	Filler Characteristics	Clinical Considerations
Microfill	40–50 nm particles	Excellent esthetics, highly polishable, yet lack in strength
Microhybrid	0.4–1.0 μm particles	High strength and good wear resistance
Nanohybrid	Conventional fillers (0.4–0.5 μm), with added nanometer-sized particles	High strength, esthetics, and polishability
Nanofill	1–100 nm particles	
Single shade	"Structural coloration" or "adaptive light matching concept"	Indicated for monochromatic teeth—not used with dark underlying structure. Simplifies color-matching procedure, restoration blends with surrounding tooth structure
Bulk-fill base	Lower filler content	Can be placed in 4–5 mm increments. Low viscosity Lower wear resistance—needs to be capped
Bulk-fill body	Higher filler content	Can be placed in 4–5 mm increments. Decreased procedure time and technique sensitivity, eliminates incremental placement and possibility of voids
Fiber reinforced	Randomly oriented E-glass fibers and particulate fillers	Used as a bulk-base in high stress-bearing situations

Microfilled resin composites
Microfilled resin composites have the advantage of high polishability and esthetic appearance, yet they lack in strength and demonstrate high polymerization shrinkage.[12] These resins may be used in low stress-bearing clinical situations that present with high esthetic demands, such as class III and class V restorations.[12,15]

Microhybrid resin composites
Microhybrid resin composites are known as "universal" composites. They have high strength, good wear resistance, and acceptable mechanical properties.[4,12] They have less polishability than microfilled composites, and surface luster may be reduced over time.[12] Microhybrid composites are indicated for most anterior applications including class IV restorations, which generally present a unique challenge due to a decrease in mechanical retention and increased stress generated through the incisal edge.[16,17]

Nanocomposites
Nanocomposites are manufactured using nanotechnology, which may greatly improve material properties.[12] They have comparable strength to microhybrids while possessing the esthetic appearance and high polishability of microfilled resins[12,18] (**Fig. 1**). There are 2 distinct types of nanocomposites: nanofilled and nanohybrid. Nanofilled composites use nanoparticles in the 1 to 100 nm range. Nanohybrids are technically hybrid composites as they combine conventional fillers (0.4–0.5 μm) with added nanometer-sized particles.[12,14]

Table 2
Clinical indications for different composite types

Composite Type	Class I	Class II	Class III	Class IV	Class V
Microfill			✓		✓
Microhybrid	✓	✓	✓	✓	✓
Nanocomposites (nanohybrid/nanofill)	✓	✓	✓	✓	
Single shade			✓		✓
Bulk-fill base	✓	✓			
Bulk-fill body	✓	✓			
Fiber reinforced		✓			

Nanocomposites have clinical performance that is comparable to microhybrid composites.[18] They do not present significant advantage in strength or hardness in comparison to microhybrids, but demonstrate comparable wear, and have actually been reported to show higher sorption and solubility values compared with microhybrids.[18] All this evidence demonstrates that nanocomposites may be used in the same clinical situations as microhybrid composites.

A meta-analysis on the clinical effectiveness of anterior restorations reported success rates of class III and class IV restorations as 95% and 90%, respectively, at 10 years, with bulk fractures being the main reason for class IV restoration failure.[19] It has, therefore, been suggested that class IV restorations require a material with higher strength than class III restorations. A recent 5-year randomized control trial compared the clinical performance of a nanofilled composite to a nanohybrid composite for class IV restorations using a split-mouth design. The study did not demonstrate a significant difference between the 2 materials in any of the outcome measures.[14]

Single-shade (one-shade)/limited shade composites

For an anterior composite resin to achieve clinical success, it must blend seamlessly with the surrounding tooth structure (also referred to as "chameleon effect").[20] Historically, clinicians have used multilayering techniques to create an acceptable esthetic result.[21] These techniques are time-consuming and require excellent technical skills and precise shade matching.[22] To reduce treatment complexity and technical

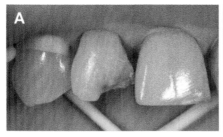
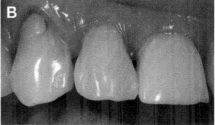

Fig. 1. Class IV restoration on maxillary right lateral incisor using the single layer technique with Filtek Supreme (3M)TM nanofilled composite resin. (*A*) Preoperative clinical presentation. (*B*) Final restoration. (Dr. Hidehiko Watanabe, Oregon Health & Science University.)

sensitivity of anterior composites, single-shade (or "one-shade") composites were developed, which are designed to esthetically simulate all shades with one nominal shade.[20]

Different manufacturers have developed one-shade universal resin composites using different technologies. According to the manufacturer, Omnichroma (Tokuama Dental America, Encinitas, CA, USA) does not contain pigments, and its optical properties rely on the concept of structural color, which is based on the optical concepts of diffraction, interference, and scattering[23] (**Fig. 2**). Another manufacturer (Venus Pearl One and Venus Diamond One: Kulzer, South Bend, IN, USA) uses "the adaptive light matching concept," where the shade of the restoration is created by the absorption of the wavelengths that are reflected by the surrounding tooth structure. From a clinical aspect, the aforementioned mechanisms used in single-shade composites that use light transmission to achieve the chameleon effect may pose a challenge in cases where masking of an underlying dark substructure is necessary.

The color-matching properties of one-shade composites has been evaluated in vitro and has shown to be promising.[24–27] Although these materials show potential to simplify color-matching procedures, clinical studies are needed to assess their esthetic performance in the intraoral environment.

Resin-Based Composites for Posterior Direct Restorations

Posterior restorations experience different challenges than anterior restorations. The demand for high esthetics is replaced with a need for high strength, due to the increased load bearing requirements of posterior restorations. Microhybrid composites and nanocomposites are generally considered the materials of choice for the posterior region, specifically those with formulations containing at least 60% filler by volume.[5] These materials are often placed using incremental techniques, which were developed to minimize polymerization shrinkage and ensure adequate depth of cure.[5]

Nanocomposites

A systematic review of randomized clinical trials comparing the clinical performance of nanocomposites (nanofilled/nanohybrid) to microhybrid composites demonstrated comparable clinical effectiveness for both types of composites for posterior applications.[28] Nanocomposites did not seem to be superior to microhybrid composites in terms of surface characteristics, marginal quality, or resistance to wear. Therefore, material choice is based on operator preference.

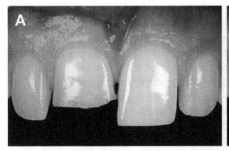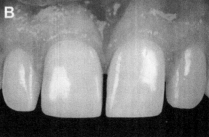

Fig. 2. Class IV restoration on maxillary right central incisor using single-shade Omnichroma (Tokuyama). (*A*) Preoperative clinical presentation. (*B*) Final restoration. (Clinical work and photographs: Dr. Marcos A. Vargas, University of Iowa (with written permission).)

Bulk-fill composites

Bulk-fill composites were developed to increase depth of cure and allow for higher efficiency in posterior restorations. These materials present an alternative to the incremental placement technique, which can be time-consuming and may also create voids from air entrapment between increments.[29] The composition of different bulk-fills varies considerably.[30] These composites are formulated with either increased concentration of reactive photoinitiators, inclusion of monomers that act as modulators, reduction in filler loading, and/or an increase in translucency.[31]

There are 2 main categories of bulk-fills: bases and full-body bulk-fill composites.[32] The base (also referred to as flowable) bulk-fill composites are low viscosity and have lower filler content, which facilitates flow and adaptation to the cavity walls, especially important in difficult to access preparations.[30] Flowable formulations are less wear resistant and require capping with a conventional composite (also referred to as the "two-step technique").[29,30] Full-body bulk-fills have higher filler loads and paste-like consistency. These composites can be placed in one increment (up to 4–5 mm), also known as the "bulk technique."[29,30] There is one subcategory of a full-body bulk-fill manufactured by Kerr (SonicFill), which uses an air-driven handpiece and sonic vibration to decrease the material viscosity, facilitating placement (Kerr: Brea, CA, USA).

The ease of use of these materials is very appealing to the clinician but do they perform as well as conventional composites? Several systematic reviews have attempted to address this question. Arbildo-Vega and colleagues[29] examined 16 randomized clinical trials and concluded that there is no difference in the clinical performance of conventional and bulk-fill resins, regardless of type of restoration, type of tooth restored, and restoration technique. Veloso and colleagues[33] conducted a systematic review and meta-analysis of 10 studies including 941 restorations and concluded there was no statistically significant difference in the failure rates between conventional and base/flowable or full-body bulk-fill resin composite restorations. Cidreira Boaro and colleagues[34] analyzed 11 randomized clinical trials with a follow-up period up to 10 years and concluded that the clinical performance of bulk-fill and conventional composites was similar.

The last question regarding bulk-fill composites is whether these materials actually save the clinician chairside time. On a systematic review and meta-analysis, Bellinaso and colleagues[35] concluded that full-body bulk-fill composites require less time than conventional resins that are placed incrementally but there is not enough data to make the same conclusion for flowable bulk-fill.[35]

Fiber-reinforced composites

Short fiber-reinforced composites (SFRCs) were developed to increase stress absorption and increase fracture toughness, with the intended use as a bulk base in high stress-bearing posterior restorations.[36] These composites consist of randomly oriented E-glass fibers, particulate fillers, and a resin matrix.[37] It is suggested that these materials should be recommended as a treatment option for large and deep class I and class II cavities.[36] A recent literature review suggested that combining SFRC as a bulk base with a conventional composite cap may improve the load-bearing capacity of the restoration but this review was limited to in vitro studies.[36] There are different formulations of SFRCs, and comparative studies have shown different physical properties, with everX Flow demonstrating superior fracture toughness and good wear resistance.[38,39] Other studies support the theory that SFRCs can significantly reinforce flowable composite resins and improve their physical properties in high stress-bearing restorations.[38–40]

A few studies have compared the use of SFRC to indirect composite restorations. One in-vitro study compared direct restorations using everX Flow base with a layer of conventional composite to indirect composite inlays for large mesial-occlusal-distal (MOD) preparations.[41] In this study, the direct SFRCs performed as well as the indirect composite inlays. One randomized clinical trial comparing SFRCs to resin composite onlays for complex molar restorations demonstrated acceptable clinical performance at 1 year follow-up.[42] Although these studies show high potential for SFRCs for large posterior direct restorations, more clinical trials are needed to further assess their clinical performance.

RESIN-BASED COMPOSITES FOR INDIRECT RESTORATIONS

Indirect composite restorations are considered a minimally invasive option and have been used for many years as an alternative to direct composites.[43,44] Restoring a tooth with composite resin using the indirect technique implies capturing an impression of the prepared tooth and fabricating the restoration using composite resin material extraorally[45] (**Fig. 3**). The restoration is subsequently bonded intraorally using an appropriate luting agent.[45,46] Compared with direct composite restorations, indirect composites result in improved physical and mechanical properties, easier development of ideal contours and anatomy, and better control on developing occlusal and proximal contacts, although also allowing for easier intraoral repair.[43,45,47] Additionally, because polymerization shrinkage does not occur intraorally, they exhibit less marginal leakage over time,[43] which is the most common reason for failure of a direct composite restoration.[6] However, indirect composites require more steps for their fabrication, are more expensive than direct composites, and lead to removal of additional tooth structure to ensure path of insertion.[43,45]

High Temperature/High Pressure Processed Resin-Based Composites

Resin-based composites for indirect applications essentially use the same technology as direct composites,[44] which is a composite resin matrix [bisphenol A-glycidyl methacrylate (BisGMA), triethylene glycol dimethacrylate (TEGDMA), ethylene glycol dimethacrylate (EDMA), ethyl methacrylate (EMA), or urethane dimethacrylate (UDMA)] with various silica or ceramic fillers.[48] Indirect composites also incorporate other formulation enhancements such as fibers or matrix modifications that further improve their physical properties.[44] The main difference compared with direct composites is that indirect materials are cured in the laboratory, using an additional postcure processing, such as the use of high temperature (HT, 180°–200°C) and/or high pressure (HP, 250–300 MPa), under nitrogen atmosphere in a curing chamber.[47,49] These HT/HP-polymerized resins exhibit higher degree of conversion, greater filler volume, and higher matrix density compared with direct composites that are polymerized intraorally using light curing only.[6,43,50] Consequently, they exhibit significantly improved flexural strength, Weibull modulus, hardness and density compared with photopolymerized resins.[47]

Resin-Based CAD/CAM Composites

Resin-based Computer-aided design Computer-aided manufacturing (CAD/CAM) composites were first introduced in 2001 by 3M (Paradigm MZ100; 3M Espe; St Paul, MN, USA), which resulted from the factory processing of the same company's successful direct composite material (Z100; 3M Espe; St Paul, MN, USA).[47,51] Multiple products have entered the market since then,[47] and new, enhanced formulations are being developed rapidly.[52] These materials, often referred to as "particle-filled

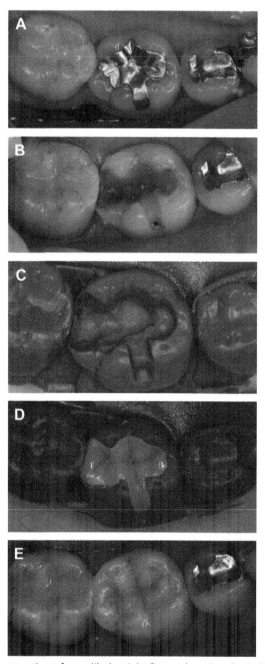

Fig. 3. Composite restoration of mandibular right first molar using the indirect technique. (*A*) Preoperative clinical presentation with a large occlusal amalgam. (*B*) Tooth prepared for indirect composite restoration. (*C*) Working model fabricated with Impregum (3M) TM from a polyvinyl siloxane impression (not pictured). (*D*) Completed indirect composite restoration. The restoration was fabricated and cured chairside with a layering technique using Estelite Omega: Tokuyama, Dental America: Encinitas, CA, USA. TM and Clearfil Majesty Flow: Kuraray Noritake; New York, NY, USA. TM. (*E*) Final indirect composite restoration, bonded to tooth. (Clinical work and photographs: Dr. Hidehiko Watanabe, Oregon Health and Sciences University.)

composites," generally consist of a composite resin polymer matrix with embedded ceramic-based or silica particles acting as fillers.[53] The composition and relative percentages of the matrix and ceramic fillers varies among different materials and significantly affects the mechanical and physical properties of the final product. Filler percentage among the most commonly used CAD/CAM composite blocks ranges from about 70% (Cerasmart; GC Corporation, Tokyo Japan) to almost 80% (Lava Ultimate; 3M Espe; St Paul, MN, USA). In 2013, Vita introduced Enamic, a resin-based composite material consisting of a presintered, resin-infiltrated ceramic network with high filler volume and, therefore, better mechanical properties.[47] Compared with ceramics, resin-based CAD/CAM composites exhibit less crack formation during their manufacturing process,[54] better marginal integrity postmilling,[55] and are easier to adjust and repair.[50] As with any composite material, adhesive bonding protocols are indicated when using these products.[55]

Three-Dimensional-Printable Resin-Based Composites

Currently, there are few composite materials available for additive manufacturing three-dimensional (3D printing) of indirect restorations using digital light processing or stereolithographic technology.[53] A prerequisite for successful completion of the 3D printing process is maintaining a stable liquid consistency of the material[56,57]; for composite-based materials, achieving such consistency essentially translates to less inorganic filler content compared with traditional CAD CAM composite blocks.[56] Less filler content subsequently lessens material stiffness[56] and flexural modulus[56] and poses a challenge in material handling.[58] These printable resin-based composites are still emerging, and the lack of data regarding their clinical performance does not enable any evidence-based recommendations for their clinical use at this point. Early reports suggest that their high stain susceptibility precludes their long-term use as restorative materials.[59]

Clinical Applications of Indirect Resin-Based Composites

Large posterior restorations

Recent systematic reviews have not shown significant difference in the long-term performance of direct and indirect composite restorations,[43,45] and both treatment approaches seem to have comparable clinical longevity.[6] To date, there are no clear guidelines in regards to selection of the appropriate treatment protocol (direct vs indirect), which remains largely subjective and dependent on operator preference and/or experience.[45] An indirect approach may be more practical in the following cases:

- When the isthmus width exceeds two-thirds of the distance between the buccal and lingual cusp tips, rendering cuspal coverage more appropriate,[6]
- When matrix adaptation is compromised due to tooth positioning (posing a challenge in establishing an ideal proximal contact), and
- When the patient cannot open wide for the time that is needed to complete a large direct restoration (due to temporomandibular joint [TMJ] pathosis or other conditions affecting mouth opening, such as scleroderma).

When compared with ceramic restorations (partial or full coverage), indirect composite restorations are less expensive and cause significantly less wear to the opposing dentition compared with ceramic crowns.[55] There is currently a lack of well-controlled long-term clinical studies comparing indirect posterior restorations using ceramic versus composite materials; therefore, any definitive conclusions about their clinical performance cannot be made, and selection of the appropriate treatment approach remains case-dependent.[60]

Both success and survival rates of indirect composite posterior onlays have been reported to be lower than those of ceramic onlays.[60] The most common complications that have been reported for composite onlays are similar in nature to those reported for direct composite restorations, namely marginal breakdown and leakage, secondary caries, wear, and fracture.[46] However, indirect composite onlays still present reasonable 10-year survival rate of 80% or more, rendering them a valid treatment option for large posterior restorations when finances are a concern[60] (**Fig. 4**).

Full coverage restorations (crowns)

Highly translucent ceramics are widely accepted as the most esthetic and durable crown material option. However, these restorations are also associated with high cost, risk of chipping or fracture, and lack of predictable reparability.[47] Composite materials have been proposed as a low-cost alternative crown material but evidence about their long-term performance is not nearly as robust as it is for ceramics. A 24-month clinical assessment of composite CAD/CAM crowns[55] indicated a success rate of 95% at 1 year and 85.7% at 2 years, whereas failure rate was 5% at 2 years. Anatomic form and marginal adaptation were the clinical parameters that exhibited the highest degree of deterioration over time, and the authors stressed the importance of following strict bonding protocols to optimize success for this type of restorations. Another laboratory study comparing full coverage restorations fabricated with either particle-filled composite blocks or ceramic blocks showed superior performance of particle-filled composites for minimum thickness restorations.[53] However, the lack of control for clinical parameters and specifically the effect of the adhesive interface was a limitation of the study, not allowing for making any clinical recommendations based on these results alone.

Under physiologic function, composite-based crowns seem to withstand occlusal forces reasonably well. However, it has been found that under lateral forces, they exhibit higher stress on their intaglio surface, making their use questionable for patients with a significant component of lateral forces, such as bruxers.[50]

Veneers

Use of indirect composites as a laminate veneer material is not yet adequately supported by literature. A survival analysis of ceramic and indirect composite

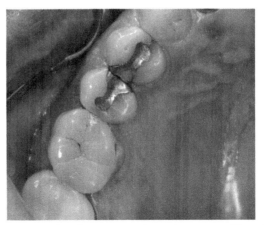

Fig. 4. Clinical appearance of indirect composite onlay on maxillary first molar (distal-occlusal-lingual [DOL]), greater than 10 years postinsertion.

(heatpolymerized and photopolymerized) laminate veneers resulted in a cumulative survival rate of 100% and 75%, respectively.[61] All failures were due to either debonding or fracture of the composite veneers. Generally, clinical parameters such as color match, surface roughness, restoration fracture, and restoration wear have been shown to be inferior for indirect composite veneers when compared with ceramic veneers.[61,62] Having these reported outcomes in mind, it can be argued that indirect composite veneers would be indicated in very limited clinical scenarios, such as the following:

- Need for reduced treatment costs
- Long-term provisional/interim treatment, with a plan for eventual replacement with ceramic material.

When choosing this approach, patients should be informed of the higher risk for future esthetic or mechanical complications and/or failures.

Multiple-unit prostheses (fixed partial dentures)
The introduction of new materials and the rapid advancements in additive manufacturing have extended the scope of proposed applications for resin-based materials, including their potential use for multiple-unit restorations replacing missing teeth. A recent laboratory study showed promising results for 3D printed 3-unit fixed partial dentures (FPDs) extending to the second premolar using a composite-based material,[63] with all prostheses being able to successfully withstand physiologic occlusal loads. However, the lack of clinical studies assessing the intraoral performance of composite-based multiple-unit prostheses renders them unsuitable for use in clinical practice.

CURRENT ADVANCES IN RESIN-BASED COMPOSITE MATERIALS

Even with the laudable progress made in resin-based materials in the last years,[64,65] as shown in the previous sections, the life span of restorations using these materials remains limited, with bacterial recolonization and fractures strongly associated to this outcome.[66] Therefore, researchers are currently focused on the development of polymeric materials with low polymerization stress and high toughness, resistance to hydrolytic and enzymatic degradation, capability of killing or inhibiting bacterial biofilm, and autonomic crack healing repairability, in order to maximize the clinical survival of the adhesive dental restorations.

Advances Leading to Improved Seal and Toughness

An important current goal for the development of dental resin composites is to mitigate the formation of microcracks at the restorative material–dental tissue interface by reducing the photopolymerization stress and to make the dental polymers more resistant to fracture by increasing their toughness.[67–69] It is important to highlight that although there is no direct evidence showing that the contraction stress generation in dental composites is associated with limited clinical life span of the dental restorations, numerous in vitro studies have provided indirect evidence that controlling polymerization stress and their effects is clinically relevant.[3] Therefore, polymeric additives have been developed and incorporated into dental composite formulations to improve the quality of the bond and marginal seal.[67–69] Among the additives, thiourethanes— synthesized via a click reaction between multifunctional thiols and isocyanates— emerged as a promising option.[9,11,67,70] These oligomers were initially incorporated into the organic matrix of methacrylate-based composites and, due to chain-transfer reactions between the pendant thiols and the polymerizing methacrylates, led to slower rates of polymerization, delayed gel/vitrification, and the formation of a more homogenous polymeric network.[67,70] These improvements into the polymerization reaction and cross-linked networks were translated in stress polymerization reduction up to 44% and fracture toughness increase up to 140%.[67] However, a common effect of the replacement of part of the organic matrix with these prepolymerized thiourethane oligomers is the overall increase in composite viscosity, which can limit the percentage of inorganic filler to be incorporated into the formulations as well as compromise the clinical handling characteristics. One strategy to overcome this drawback is to graft thiourethane oligomers to the filler particle surface rather than incorporate them directly into the organic matrix, which led to toughening and stress-reducing effects without affecting the final viscosity of the composite.[11] Recently, observations related to the stress relaxation kinetics in thiourethane-containing composites have added to the chain-transfer reactions and the formation of urethane bonds as the mechanisms responsible for these achievements and indicated that thiourethanes may be dynamic networks.[9]

The grafting of polymer brushes on inorganic filler surface has also been explored in another study and was found to be a feasible strategy to reduce shrinkage stress.[71] The incorporation of γ-methacryloxypropyltrimethoxysilane polymer brush functionalized fillers in dental composites at 30 wt% led to a 30% reduction in shrinkage stress in comparison to the control, without compromising the final conversion or the mechanical properties.[71]

Other current trends to mitigate the polymerization stress in resin-based dental composites include the development of alternative low-shrinkage comonomers.[72–74] The replacement of BisGMA with a newly synthesized diurethane dimethacrylate (2-hydroxy-1-ethyl methacrylate) in UDMA-based dental composites resulted in polymerization stress reduction between 30% and 50% and optimized water stability without jeopardizing the mechanical properties.[72] Resin composites with 50% lower polymerization stress were also formulated by the replacement of TEGDMA with a novel diallyl carbonate compound (allyl(2-(2-(((allyloxy)carbonyl)oxy)benzoyl)-5-methoxyphenyl) carbonate) in copolymerizations with BisGMA.[73] These results were achieved without compromising the final degree of conversion or the mechanical properties.[73] The copolymerization of UDMA and an ether-based compound (triethylene glycol divinylbenzyl ether) seems to also be a promising approach to modulate the polymerization reaction and, ultimately, decrease the generated stress up to 52% and increase the toughness up to 27% in comparison to the BisGMA/TEGDMA control.[74] These findings may contribute to the development of restorative materials with optimized clinical performance, which will affect the field because recent studies have demonstrated that so-called low-stress commercial composite did not improve significantly dental restorations longevity compared with conventional materials.[75–77]

Mechanical strength reinforcement has also been achieved by the design of interpenetrating polymer networks (IPNs) derived from acrylate-functionalized nanogels dispersed and polyurethane matrix.[78] This strategy provided significantly toughened polymeric networks with shape memory capability and no detrimental effects on the bulk modulus or strength in IPNs containing up to 20 wt% of nanogels.[78]

Advances Leading to Degradation Resistance

Because the limited clinical lifetime of methacrylate-based dental restorations is also strongly associated to the susceptibility of the ester bonds to hydrolytic and enzymatic degradation,[79] more stable chemical compounds have been developed and investigated as potential alternatives to the traditional formulations. Triphenyl ethane-centered ether-linked triazides were designed as ester-free hydrophobic compounds and compared with BISGMA/TEGDMA polymers.[80] In general, the ether-based systems showed significantly higher water stability than the methacrylate control (water solubility 2.3 vs 4.4 $\mu g/mm^3$) in addition to the reduced polymerization stress (0.56 vs 1.0 MPa) and enhanced flexural toughness (7.6 vs 1.6 MJ/m^3). Another tested approach was the incorporation of styrene-co-divinylbenzene nanogels into conventional dimethacrylate systems.[81] Dramatic reduction in water uptake and improved shielding throughout the bulk methacrylate-bad polymers were noticed in formulations containing the hydrophobic all-hydrocarbon nanogels at 50 wt%.[81] The hydrolytically stable approaches have also been aimed at the adhesive interface, and in combination with thiourethane-based composites, they have led to superior marginal preservation in restorations tested under clinical mimic conditions.[82]

Advances Leading to Antimicrobial Activity

Resin-based restorative surfaces are prone to biofilm formation and accumulation, which contributes to the development of secondary caries and decreased longevity of the dental restorations.[83] In an attempt to overcome this issue, researchers have focused on the development of polymeric networks containing chemically bound antibacterial agents. Quaternary ammonium compounds functionalized with hydrolytically stable acrylamides or (meth)acrylamides were synthesized and incorporated into dental composite formulations, leading to decreased biofilm formation by more than 2 orders of magnitude, higher resistance to hydrolytic degradation, and similar biocompatibility to the BisGMA/TEGDMA control group.[11] Nonsoluble quaternary ammonium has also been covalently bound to the surface of inorganic fillers and the particles (quaternary ammonium silane [QASi]) incorporated into the dental restorative materials.[84] The commercially available composite, Infinix (Nobio Ltd: Kadima, Israel), claims to be effective against multiple bacterial strains and fungi pathogens.[84]

Alternating antimicrobial/antifouling, pH-responsive, carboxybetaine-based compounds have also been developed.[85] These compounds are antifouling at neutral pH and thus prevent biofilm colonization at the resin-based surfaces. As the pH becomes acidic, the backbone of the compound is rearranged and the polymer acts as an antimicrobial agent.[85] Another emergent strategy is the incorporation of graphene-based compounds into dental restorative materials, which is facilitated by their biocompatibility, versatility, relatively simple chemical functionalization, and potent antimicrobial effect.[86,87] Graphene-containing dental polymers have shown broad antibacterial spectrum while maintaining bulk mechanical properties.[86,87] Because a potential limitation for the application of graphene in dental restorative materials may be its grayish shade, white-colored fluorinated graphene was synthesized and showed similar properties.[88]

Advances Leading to Self-Reparability

Catastrophic fracture of resin-based restorations in the oral cavity is strongly related to the formation and propagation of internal microcracks caused by masticatory forces.[89] An appealing strategy to overcome this shortcoming lies in the development of polymeric networks with self-healing properties. Extrinsic and intrinsic approaches aiming to inhibit the crack propagation and rebuild the damage have been developed.[90] The most common extrinsic strategy is based on the addition of microcapsules containing a low viscosity healing agent compound and an amine into the organic matrix.[7,8] In summary, as the cracks propagate, the capsules are ruptured and the healing agent flows into the cracked area to form covalent cross-linked bonds with the organic matrix.[91] The most popular system developed in dentistry is based on the encapsulation of TEGDMA and the amine DHEPT (N,N-dihydroxyethyl-p-toluidine) in (poly)urea formaldehyde shells.[7,8] In this system, the redox polymerization reaction is triggered by the benzoyl peroxide (BPO) dispersed into the organic matrix. The results showed healing efficiency of around 65% in polymeric systems containing 10 wt % of microcapsules while the bulk mechanical properties were maintained.[7,8] Systems composed of silica microcapsules loaded with polyacrylic acid and dispersed into an organic matrix containing fluoroaluminasilicate glass powder were also synthesized and showed healing capability of up to 25% in systems containing 5 wt% of microcapsules.[92,93]

The microvascular extrinsic approach is the most complex to be translated to dental materials applications.[90] However, given the substantial growth and progressive expansion of digital dentistry, printing prostheses and indirect restorations in the dental offices is now close to being feasible, and it may represent a driving force for the expansion of these systems.

In intrinsic self-healing dental polymers, latent functionalities within the polymeric structure (chemically or compositionally tuned) are capable of undergoing reversible chemical bonds in response to a wide variety of stimuli. Although it is challenging to ensure chemical group accessibility in a hindered cross-linked polymeric network and develop feasible manufacturing methods, they are elegant strategies that, if properly adapted and implemented to the harsh oral environment, can initiate a new generation of self-healing dental polymers. Some advancements have also been achieved with the design of urease-aided self-healing dental composites.[94,95] In this proof-of-concept system, microcracks seem to get efficiently sealed with calcium carbonate that is formed as the urease breaks down the salivary urea and binds with calcium.[94,95]

FUTURE ADVANCES: MULTIFUNCTIONAL STIMULI-RESPONSIVE DENTAL MATERIALS

The envisioned next generation of resin-based restorative dental materials is based on polymers that do not simply inertly fill a prepared cavity but rather are capable of interacting dynamically with the host environment and adapting to it. It is expected that the restorative materials will be biomimetic and stimuli-responsive, capable of retaining a set of specifically coded instructions by virtue of their chemical structure, enabling them to interact with the oral environment and perform a desired function on demand.

The dental materials field is moving toward the development of organic compounds capable of mimicking species-specific virulence factors to inhibit dysbiotic bacterial biofilm formation and promote ecological symbiosis among the oral microflora rather than broad spectrum antimicrobial effects, promoting dental tissues preservation and regeneration, and responding to the generation of mechanical stresses adapting and self-repairing.

In summary, the mission of the field is the development of multifunctional polymeric materials that can be used in preventive and treatment strategies and are able to improve oral health for individuals across their life span.

CLINICS CARE POINTS

- Microhybrid resin composites and nanocomposites exhibit both strength and esthetics, and can be used universally for both anterior and posterior restorations.
- Bulk-fill resin composites used in posterior restorations can decrease technique sensitivity and chairside time without compromising mechanical properties.
- Single-shade resin composites can simplify the process of shade selection for anterior restorations, but are best suited for smaller restorations and monochromatic teeth.

- Indirect resin composites exhibit improved physical and mechanical properties compared to direct composites, and allow for easier development of contours and anatomy for larger restorations, offering a cost-effective alternative to traditional indirect ceramic-based restorations

- Composite resin CAD/CAM materials can be an alternative option for full coverage restorations, but are still not indicated for patients exhibiting high occlusal forces.

- For the next generation of resin composites, materials may be capable of interacting actively with the host environment and adapt to it, which could subsequently be translated to dental restorations with a longer clinical lifespan.

REFERENCES

1. Bayne SC, Ferracane JL, Marshall GW, et al. The Evolution of Dental Materials over the Past Century: Silver and Gold to Tooth Color and Beyond. J Dent Res 2019;98(3):257–65.
2. Heintze SD, Rousson V. Clinical effectiveness of direct class II restorations - a meta-analysis. J Adhes Dent 2012;14(5):407–31.
3. Ferracane JL, Hilton TJ. Polymerization stress–is it clinically meaningful? Dent Mater 2016;32(1):1–10.
4. Ferracane JL. Resin composite–state of the art. Dent Mater 2011;27(1):29–38.
5. Lynch CD, Opdam NJ, Hickel R, et al. Guidance on posterior resin composites: Academy of Operative Dentistry - European Section. J Dent 2014;42(4): 377–83.
6. da Veiga AM, Cunha AC, Ferreira DM, et al. Longevity of direct and indirect resin composite restorations in permanent posterior teeth: A systematic review and meta-analysis. J Dent 2016;54:1–12.
7. Wu J, Weir MD, Melo MAS, et al. Effects of water-aging on self-healing dental composite containing microcapsules. J dentistry 2016;47:86–93.
8. Wu J, Weir MD, Zhang Q, et al. Novel self-healing dental resin with microcapsules of polymerizable triethylene glycol dimethacrylate and N, N-dihydroxyethyl-p-toluidine. Dental Mater 2016;32(2):294–304.
9. Fugolin A, Costa A, Lewis S, et al. Probing stress relaxation behavior in glassy methacrylate networks containing thio-carbamate additives. J Mater Chem B 2021;9(13):3015–24.
10. Fugolin AP, Dobson A, Huynh V, et al. Antibacterial, ester-free monomers: Polymerization kinetics, mechanical properties, biocompatibility and anti-biofilm activity. Acta Biomater 2019;100:132–41.
11. Fugolin AP, Sundfeld D, Ferracane JL, et al. Toughening of dental composites with thiourethane-modified filler interfaces. Sci Rep 2019;9(1):1–9.
12. Sakaguchi RLFJ, Powers JM. Craig's restorative dental materials. 14th edition. Missouri: Elsevier Mosby; 2018. p. 352.
13. Vargas MA, Margeas R. A systematic approach to contouring and polishing anterior resin composite restorations: A checklist manifesto. J Esthet Restor Dent 2021;33(1):20–6.
14. Demirci M, Tuncer S, Sancakli HS, et al. Five-year Clinical Evaluation of a Nanofilled and a Nanohybrid Composite in Class IV Cavities. Oper Dent 2018;43(3): 261–71.
15. Dietschi D, Shahidi C, Krejci I. Clinical performance of direct anterior composite restorations: a systematic literature review and critical appraisal. Int J Esthet Dent 2019;14(3):252–70.

16. Demarco FF, Collares K, Coelho-de-Souza FH, et al. Anterior composite restorations: A systematic review on long-term survival and reasons for failure. Dent Mater 2015;31(10):1214–24.

17. Moura FR, Romano AR, Lund RG, et al. Three-year clinical performance of composite restorations placed by undergraduate dental students. Braz Dent J 2011; 22(2):111–6.

18. Alzraikat H, Burrow MF, Maghaireh GA, et al. Nanofilled Resin Composite Properties and Clinical Performance: A Review. Oper Dent 2018;43(4):E173.e90.

19. Heintze SD, Rousson V, Hickel R. Clinical effectiveness of direct anterior restorations–a meta-analysis. Dent Mater 2015;31(5):481–95.

20. Lucena C, Ruiz-López J, Pulgar R, et al. Optical behavior of one-shaded resin-based composites. Dent Mater 2021;37(5):840–8.

21. Dietschi D, Fahl N Jr. Shading concepts and layering techniques to master direct anterior composite restorations: an update. Br Dent J 2016;221(12):765–71.

22. Iyer RS, Babani VR, Yaman P, et al. Color match using instrumental and visual methods for single, group, and multi-shade composite resins. J Esthet Restor Dent 2021;33(2):394–400.

23. Dumanli AG, Savin T. Recent advances in the biomimicry of structural colours. Chem Soc Rev 2016;45(24):6698–724.

24. de Abreu JLB, Sampaio CS, Benalcázar Jalkh EB, et al. Analysis of the color matching of universal resin composites in anterior restorations. J Esthet Restor Dent 2021;33(2):269–76.

25. Saegusa M, Kurokawa H, Takahashi N, et al. Evaluation of Color-matching Ability of a Structural Colored Resin Composite. Oper Dent 2021;46(3):306–15.

26. Pereira Sanchez N, Powers JM, Paravina RD. Instrumental and visual evaluation of the color adjustment potential of resin composites. J Esthet Restor Dent 2019; 31(5):465–70.

27. Kobayashi S, Nakajima M, Furusawa K, et al. Color adjustment potential of single-shade resin composite to various-shade human teeth: Effect of structural color phenomenon. Dent Mater J 2021;40(4):1033–40.

28. Angerame D, De Biasi M. Do Nanofilled/Nanohybrid Composites Allow for Better Clinical Performance of Direct Restorations Than Traditional Microhybrid Composites? A Systematic Review. Oper Dent 2018;43(4):E191–209.

29. Arbildo-Vega HI, Lapinska B, Panda S, et al. Clinical Effectiveness of Bulk-Fill and Conventional Resin Composite Restorations: Systematic Review and Meta-Analysis. Polymers (Basel) 2020;12(8):1786.

30. Van Ende A, De Munck J, Lise DP, et al. Bulk-Fill Composites: A Review of the Current Literature. J Adhes Dent 2017;19(2):95–109.

31. Fronza BM, Rueggeberg FA, Braga RR, et al. Monomer conversion, microhardness, internal marginal adaptation, and shrinkage stress of bulk-fill resin composites. Dent Mater 2015;31(12):1542–51.

32. Chesterman J, Jowett A, Gallacher A, et al. Bulk-fill resin-based composite restorative materials: a review. Br Dent J 2017;222(5):337–44.

33. Veloso SRM, Lemos CAA, de Moraes SLD, et al. Clinical performance of bulk-fill and conventional resin composite restorations in posterior teeth: a systematic review and meta-analysis. Clin Oral Investig 2019;23(1):221–33.

34. Cidreira Boaro LC, Pereira Lopes D, de Souza ASC, et al. Clinical performance and chemical-physical properties of bulk fill composites resin -a systematic review and meta-analysis. Dent Mater 2019;35(10):e249–64.

35. Bellinaso MD, Soares FZM, Rocha RO. Do bulk-fill resins decrease the restorative time in posterior teeth? A systematic review and meta-analysis of in vitro studies. J Investig Clin Dent 2019;10(4):e12463.
36. Garoushi S, Gargoum A, Vallittu PK, et al. Short fiber-reinforced composite restorations: A review of the current literature. J Investig Clin Dent 2018;9(3):e12330.
37. Keulemans FGS, Lassila L. Fillings and core buildups (Book Chapter). In: Vallittu POM, editor. A clinical guide to principles of fibre reinforced composites (FRCs) in dentistry. Cambridge: Woodhead Publishing; 2018. p. 131–63.
38. Alshabib A, Silikas N, Watts DC. Hardness and fracture toughness of resin-composite materials with and without fibers. Dent Mater 2019;35(8):1194–203.
39. Lassila L, Keulemans F, Vallittu PK, et al. Characterization of restorative short-fiber reinforced dental composites. Dent Mater J 2020;39(6):992–9.
40. Lassila L, Keulemans F, Säilynoja E, et al. Mechanical properties and fracture behavior of flowable fiber reinforced composite restorations. Dent Mater 2018; 34(4):598–606.
41. Soares LM, Razaghy M, Magne P. Optimization of large MOD restorations: Composite resin inlays vs. short fiber-reinforced direct restorations. Dent Mater 2018; 34(4):587–97.
42. ElAziz RH, Mohammed MM, Gomaa HA. Clinical Performance of Short-fiber-reinforced Resin Composite Restorations vs Resin Composite Onlay Restorations in Complex Cavities of Molars (Randomized Clinical Trial). J Contemp Dent Pract 2020;21(3):296–303.
43. Azeem RA, Sureshbabu NM. Clinical performance of direct versus indirect composite restorations in posterior teeth: A systematic review. J Conserv Dent 2018; 21(1):2–9.
44. Shellard E, Duke ES. Indirect composite resin materials for posterior applications. Compend Contin Educ Dent 1999;20(12):1166–71.
45. Angeletaki F, Gkogkos A, Papazoglou E, et al. Direct versus indirect inlay/onlay composite restorations in posterior teeth. A systematic review and meta-analysis. J Dent 2016;53:12–21.
46. Derchi G, Marchio V, Borgia V, et al. Twelve-year longitudinal clinical evaluation of bonded indirect composite resin inlays. Quintessence Int 2019;50(6):448–54.
47. Ruse ND, Sadoun MJ. Resin-composite blocks for dental CAD/CAM applications. J Dent Res 2014;93(12):1232–4.
48. Mandikos MN, McGivney GP, Davis E, et al. A comparison of the wear resistance and hardness of indirect composite resins. J Prosthet Dent 2001;85(4):386–95.
49. Nguyen JF, Migonney V, Ruse ND, et al. Resin composite blocks via high-pressure high-temperature polymerization. Dent Mater 2012;28(5):529–34.
50. Duan Y, Griggs JA. Effect of elasticity on stress distribution in CAD/CAM dental crowns: Glass ceramic vs. polymer-matrix composite. J Dent 2015;43(6):742–9.
51. Rusin RP. Properties and applications of a new composite block for CAD/CAM. Compend Contin Educ Dent 2001;22(6 Suppl):35–41.
52. Ling L, Ma Y, Malyala R. A novel CAD/CAM resin composite block with high mechanical properties. Dent Mater 2021;37(7):1150–5.
53. Zimmermann M, Ender A, Egli G, et al. Fracture load of CAD/CAM-fabricated and 3D-printed composite crowns as a function of material thickness. Clin Oral Investig 2019;23(6):2777–84.
54. Moradi Z, Abbasi M, Khalesi R, et al. Fracture Toughness Comparison of Three Indirect Composite Resins Using 4-Point Flexural Strength Method. Eur J Dent 2020;14(2):212–6.

55. Zimmermann M, Koller C, Reymus M, et al. Clinical Evaluation of Indirect Particle-Filled Composite Resin CAD/CAM Partial Crowns after 24 Months. J Prosthodont 2018;27(8):694–9.
56. Grzebieluch W, Kowalewski P, Grygier D, et al. Printable and Machinable Dental Restorative Composites for CAD/CAM Application-Comparison of Mechanical Properties, Fractographic, Texture and Fractal Dimension Analysis. Materials (Basel) 2021;14(17):4919.
57. Tahayeri A, Morgan M, Fugolin AP, et al. 3D printed versus conventionally cured provisional crown and bridge dental materials. Dent Mater 2018;34(2):192–200.
58. Scotti CK, Velo M, Rizzante FAP, et al. Physical and surface properties of a 3D-printed composite resin for a digital workflow. J Prosthet Dent 2020;124(5):614.e1-5.
59. Alharbi N, Alharbi A, Osman R. Stain Susceptibility of 3D-Printed Nanohybrid Composite Restorative Material and the Efficacy of Different Stain Removal Techniques: An In Vitro Study. Materials (Basel) 2021;14(19):5621.
60. Bustamante-Hernández N, Montiel-Company JM, Bellot-Arcís C, et al. Clinical behavior of ceramic, hybrid and composite onlays. a systematic review and meta-analysis. Int J Environ Res Public Health 2020;17(20):7582.
61. Gresnigt MMM, Cune MS, Jansen K, et al. Randomized clinical trial on indirect resin composite and ceramic laminate veneers: Up to 10-year findings. J Dent 2019;86:102–9.
62. Gresnigt MM, Kalk W, Ozcan M. Randomized clinical trial of indirect resin composite and ceramic veneers: up to 3-year follow-up. J Adhes Dent 2013;15(2):181–90.
63. Corbani K, Hardan L, Eid R, et al. Fracture Resistance of Three-unit Fixed Dental Prostheses Fabricated with Milled and 3D Printed Composite-based Materials. J Contemp Dent Pract 2021;22(9):985–90.
64. Wang Y, Zhu M, Zhu X. Functional fillers for dental resin composites. Acta Biomater 2021;122:50–65.
65. Tsujimoto A, Barkmeier WW, Fischer NG, et al. Wear of resin composites: Current insights into underlying mechanisms, evaluation methods and influential factors. Jpn Dental Sci Rev 2018;54(2):76–87.
66. Collares K, Opdam NJ, Peres KG, et al. Higher experience of caries and lower income trajectory influence the quality of restorations: A multilevel analysis in a birth cohort. J dentistry 2018;68:79–84.
67. Bacchi A, Nelson M, Pfeifer CS. Characterization of methacrylate-based composites containing thio-urethane oligomers. Dental Mater 2016;32(2):233–9.
68. Fronza B, Rad I, Shah P, et al. Nanogel-based filler-matrix interphase for polymerization stress reduction. J dental Res 2019;98(7):779–85.
69. Gao G, Han X, Sowan N, et al. Stress Relaxation via Covalent Dynamic Bonds in Nanogel-Containing Thiol–Ene Resins. ACS Macro Lett 2020;9(5):713–9.
70. Bacchi A, Dobson A, Ferracane J, et al. Thio-urethanes improve properties of dual-cured composite cements. J dental Res 2014;93(12):1320–5.
71. Shah PK, Stansbury JW. Photopolymerization shrinkage-stress reduction in polymer-based dental restoratives by surface modification of fillers. Dental Mater 2021;37(4):578–87.
72. Fugolin AP, de Paula AB, Dobson A, et al. Alternative monomer for BisGMA-free resin composites formulations. Dental Mater 2020;36(7):884–92.
73. González-López JA, Pérez-Mondragón AA, Cuevas-Suárez CE, et al. Dental composite resins with low polymerization stress based on a new allyl carbonate monomer. J Mech Behav Biomed Mater 2020;110:103955.

74. Wang X, Huyang G, Palagummi SV, et al. High performance dental resin composites with hydrolytically stable monomers. Dental Mater 2018;34(2):228–37.
75. Hoseinifar R, Mortazavi-Lahijani E, Mollahassani H, et al. One year clinical evaluation of a low shrinkage composite compared with a packable composite resin: a randomized clinical trial. J Dentistry (Tehran, Iran) 2017;14(2):84.
76. Frascino S, Fagundes T, Silva U, et al. Randomized prospective clinical trial of class II restorations using low-shrinkage flowable resin composite. Oper dentistry 2020;45(1):19–29.
77. Yantcheva S. Clinical evaluation of low shrinkage resin composites in class II restorations-two years follow up. MedInform 2021;1:1269–77. https://doi.org/10.18044/MEDINFORM.202181.1269.
78. Gao G, Wang X, Chen M, et al. Functional Nanogels as a Route to Interpenetrating Polymer Networks with Improved Mechanical Properties. Macromolecules 2021;54(23):10657–66. https://doi.org/10.1021/acs.macromol.1c01242.
79. Gonzalez-Bonet A, Kaufman G, Yang Y, et al. Preparation of dental resins resistant to enzymatic and hydrolytic degradation in oral environments. Biomacromolecules 2015;16(10):3381–8.
80. Wang X, Gao G, Song HB, et al. Evaluation of a photo-initiated copper (I)-catalyzed azide-alkyne cycloaddition polymer network with improved water stability and high mechanical performance as an ester-free dental restorative. Dental Mater 2021;37(10):1592–600.
81. Rad IY, Lewis S, Barros MD, et al. Suppression of hydrolytic degradation in labile polymer networks via integrated styrenic nanogels. Dental Mater 2021;37(8):1295–306.
82. de Lucena F, Lewis S, Fugolin A, et al. Triacrylamide-based adhesives stabilize bonds in physiologic conditions. J dental Res 2022;101(6):647–54.
83. Cazzaniga G, Ottobelli M, Ionescu AC, et al. In vitro biofilm formation on resin-based composites after different finishing and polishing procedures. J dentistry 2017;67:43–52.
84. Rechmann P, Le CQ, Chaffee BW, et al. Demineralization prevention with a new antibacterial restorative composite containing QASi nanoparticles: an in situ study. Clin Oral Investig 2021;25(9):5293–305.
85. Cheng G, Cao B. Switchable antimicrobial and antifouling carboxybetaine-based hydrogels and elastomers with enhanced mechanical properties. United States: Google Patents; 2019.
86. Yousefi M, Dadashpour M, Hejazi M, et al. Anti-bacterial activity of graphene oxide as a new weapon nanomaterial to combat multidrug-resistance bacteria. Mater Sci Eng C 2017;74:568–81.
87. Radhi A, Mohamad D, Rahman FSA, et al. Mechanism and factors influence of graphene-based nanomaterials antimicrobial activities and application in dentistry. J Mater Res Technology 2021;(11):1290–307. https://doi.org/10.1016/j.jmrt.2021.01.093.
88. Sun L, Yan Z, Duan Y, et al. Improvement of the mechanical, tribological and antibacterial properties of glass ionomer cements by fluorinated graphene. Dental Mater 2018;34(6):e115–27.
89. Albakry M. Insightful Understanding of the Role of the Mechanical Properties in Defining the Reliability of All-Ceramic Dental Restorations: A Review. J Biomater Nanobiotechnology 2021;12(4):57–78.
90. Diesendruck CE, Sottos NR, Moore JS, et al. Biomimetic self-healing. Angew Chem Int Edition 2015;54(36):10428–47.

91. Mauldin TC, Kessler M. Self-healing polymers and composites. Int Mater Rev 2010;55(6):317–46.
92. Huyang G, Debertin AE, Sun J. Design and development of self-healing dental composites. Mater Des 2016;94:295–302.
93. Yahyazadehfar M, Huyang G, Wang X, et al. Durability of self-healing dental composites: A comparison of performance under monotonic and cyclic loading. Mater Sci Eng C 2018;93:1020–6.
94. Seifan M, Sarabadani Z, Berenjian A. Development of an innovative urease-aided self-healing dental composite. catalysts 2020;10(1):84.
95. Seifan M, Sarabadani Z, Berenjian A. Microbially induced calcium carbonate precipitation to design a new type of bio self-healing dental composite. Appl Microbiol Biotechnol 2020;104(5):2029–37.

Dental Light-Curing—Assessing the Blue-Light Hazard

Dayane Oliveira, DDS, MS, PhD, Mateus Garcia Rocha, DDS, MS, PhD*

KEYWORDS

- Light curing units • Photopolymerization • Blue-light hazard • Eyewear protection
- Occupational exposure

KEY POINTS

- Dental light-curing units emit high-power visible light that can cure resin materials in seconds; however, the use of high-power visible light can cause critical health issues.
- Dental personnel should be trained to use light-curing units (LCUs), and they should wear protective eye filters when operating or manipulating LCUs.
- If the use of LCUs is causing you persistent afterimages or blurred vision, you have been exposed to an excessive amount of light, and you should improve your LCU safety measures.
- The misuse of high-power LCUs can cause soft tissues burns and pulpal inflammation; however, the use of the correct radiant exposure and tooth cooling techniques (ie, increase of airflow to the tooth while curing by using an air syringe) can reduce any potential risks of using these LCUs.

INTRODUCTION

Light-curing units (LCUs) are essential for photopolymerization in modern dentistry. The basic idea is to instantly transform a liquid or viscous monomer into a solid material on light exposure inside the patient's mouth.[1] Because a photopolymerization reaction involves a photoinitiator system, a polymerizable medium (monomers), and an LCU, a strong correlation exists between them.[2]

The literature on how to properly light-cure dental materials is vast.[3] However, such devices may pose severe risks to dental personnel and patients. Therefore, the objective of the present article is to review the characteristics of the blue light emitted by LCUs, the physiology of the human eye and dental tissues to visible light, and how to efficiently use LCUs to mitigate risks and conduct proper light curing in dentistry.

Center for Dental Biomaterials, Department of Restorative Dental Sciences, University of Florida - College of Dentistry, 1395 Center Drive D9-6, Gainesville, FL 32610, USA
* Corresponding author.
E-mail address: mrocha@dental.ufl.edu

Dent Clin N Am 66 (2022) 537–550
https://doi.org/10.1016/j.cden.2022.05.004
0011-8532/22/© 2022 Elsevier Inc. All rights reserved.

dental.theclinics.com

LIGHT CURING IN DENTISTRY

Light curing in dentistry was first attempted clinically in the early 1970s using ultraviolet light (UV, about 365 nm).[4] However, this photopolymerization system did not succeed due to the harmful effects of the UV energy being exposed to human eyes (corneal burns and cataract formation), poor depth of penetration into materials, and many issues with the properties of the UV-cured dental materials.[4] In 1976, advances in visible light polymerization allowed the development of resin materials containing camphorquinone (CQ) and reducing agents (ie, tertiary amines) photopolymerized by blue light.[2,5] The advantages of using visible light revolutionized dentistry and resin-based materials are considered long-lasting treatments for restorative dentistry.[5] Because long visible wavelengths penetrate deeper into materials, the depth of cure of these materials was increased. Thus, besides improving the properties of light-cured resin materials, it also allowed a reduced chair time. The incremental technique increased from a single millimeter to now 2 to 5 mm.[4,5] Although visible light curing has reduced potential hazards for developing cataracts and macular degeneration compared with UV light curing, it still can cause direct retinal burning and retinal photochemical damage. The potential for visible light curing in dentistry to cause or contribute to macular degeneration in dental personnel over their working lifespan remains unknown.[6–8]

For many years, Quartz-Tungsten Halogen (QTH) LCUs were very popular. QTHs emit the entire visible spectral range from an incandescent light bulb, and a prism filters violet and blue light.[4] However, in 2009, the European Union and other countries began a phase-out of inefficient incandescent bulbs to widen efforts to deal with climate change.[9] In modern dentistry, light-emitting diodes (LEDs) are the most popular LCUs, as they have several advantages compared with QTH, such as portability, power efficiency, and more consistent light output.[3,4]

The first and second generations of dental LEDs, also called monowave or single peak, emit a narrow band within the blue light range (420–495 nm) with a peak around 460 nm (**Fig. 1**A).[4,10] Later, with other photoinitiator systems with absorption in different regions of the light spectrum, LED LCUs with light emission in both the violet

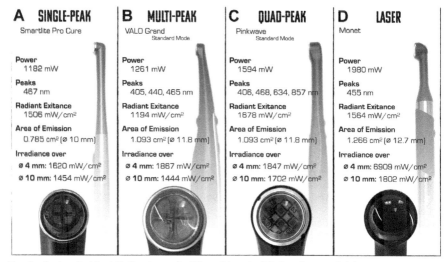

A   SINGLE-PEAK
Smartlite Pro Cure

Power
  1182 mW

Peaks
  467 nm

Radiant Exitance
  1506 mW/cm²

Area of Emission
  0.785 cm² (ø 10 mm)

Irradiance over
  ø **4 mm:** 1620 mW/cm²
  ø **10 mm:** 1454 mW/cm²

B   MULTI-PEAK
VALO Grand
  Standard Mode

Power
  1261 mW

Peaks
  405, 440, 465 nm

Radiant Exitance
  1194 mW/cm²

Area of Emission
  1.093 cm² (ø 11.8 mm)

Irradiance over
  ø **4 mm:** 1867 mW/cm²
  ø **10 mm:** 1444 mW/cm²

C   QUAD-PEAK
Pinkwave
  Standard Mode

Power
  1594 mW

Peaks
  406, 468, 634, 857 nm

Radiant Exitance
  1678 mW/cm²

Area of Emission
  1.093 cm² (ø 11.8 mm)

Irradiance over
  ø **4 mm:** 1847 mW/cm²
  ø **10 mm:** 1702 mW/cm²

D   LASER
Monet

Power
  1980 mW

Peaks
  455 nm

Radiant Exitance
  1564 mW/cm²

Area of Emission
  1.266 cm² (ø 12.7 mm)

Irradiance over
  ø **4 mm:** 6909 mW/cm²
  ø **10 mm:** 1802 mW/cm²

Fig. 1. Curing lights. (*A*) Single peak; (*B*) multipeak; (*C*) Quadwave; (*D*) laser.

(380–420 nm) and blue range were released into the market. These LCUs, also known as multiwave, polywave[a], or multipeak LCUs, are devices made up of a combination of 2 or more LED chips emitting over different wavelengths (**Fig. 1B**).[3,4,10] The multipeak LEDs emit light from 380 to 540 nm, comprising the violet and blue range. More recently, a new generation of curing lights emitting red and near-infrared (NIR) was released on the market (**Fig. 1C**). The so-called Quadwave[b] technology claims to increase the degree of conversion and reduce polymerization shrinkage. However, at the present moment, there is no scientific evidence that red and NIR lights have benefits on modern composites containing CQ or other alternative violet or blue light–absorbing photoinitiators.

Dental laser diodes were released into the market claiming to light-cure dental materials in 1s (**Fig. 1D**). Lasers (*plural for the acronym Light Amplification by Stimulated Emission of Radiation*) are distinguished from other light sources by their coherence. Laser beams have a minor divergence to concentrate their power at a great distance. Also, the narrow emission spectrum from the lasers is designed to excite the photoinitiators used within the red blood cells at their maximum absorption efficiency. Although some materials can efficiently photopolymerize in this curing condition, these lasers can be considered medical devices with a high potential to cause injuries if misused. According to the United States Food and Drug Administration (FDA) 501(k) premarket notification regulations, dental curing lasers are class II medical devices with a moderate risk of injuries. However, lasers with more than 500 mW of power are classified as high-powered Class 4 visible-beam lasers. A Class 4 laser operator should be trained by a Laser Safety Officer (LSO) with the duties and responsibilities defined in the ANSI Z136 standard published by the American National Standard Institute (ANSI).

The critical problem with visible light curing is that the wavelength needed to initiate the photoinitiator systems overlap within the frequencies known to cause photochemical and photothermal injuries to ocular, gingival, and pulp tissues.[11–13] Furthermore, contemporary light-curable materials require radiant exposure of 10 to 40 J/cm^2 to polymerize dental materials adequately.[3,14] To deliver this amount of energy in a short exposure time, the use of high-powered LCUs with a high capacity of light emission is required.[3,7,13] LCUs are considered high-powered when emitting 1000 mW/cm^2 or higher. Nowadays most LCUs on the market are considered high-powered. Despite the clinical advantage of light-activating materials in seconds, high-irradiance visible light can cause critical health issues.[7,8]

THE BLUE-LIGHT HAZARD

Exposure to blue light is very significant in modern life. Most of the population is exposed to artificial light over the entire day. Because light has a cumulative effect and its power is affected by several characteristics, such as wavelength, intensity, and duration of the exposure, it is crucial to consider the power and the spectral output of the dental LCUs to minimize the risks associated with excessive blue-light exposure.

Potential Ocular Hazards

In humans, photoreception occurs in the retina by 3 photoreceptors: cones, rods, and the intrinsically photosensitive retinal ganglion cells.[6] **Fig. 2A** shows the human eye

---

[a] Polywave is a trademark of Ivoclar Vivadent.

[b] Quadwave is a trademark of Vista Apex.

A 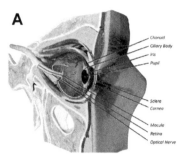 B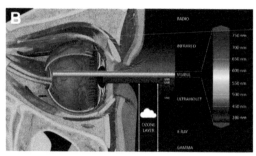

Fig. 2. (*A*) Cross-section view of the human eye anatomy. The eye is a fluid-filled sphere enclosed by 3 layers of tissue. The first layer is a tough white fibrous tissue (*Sclera*) that connects with a specialized transparent tissue (*Cornea*) that permits light to enter the eye. The second layer of tissue includes 3 distinct but continuous structures: the *Iris*, the *Ciliary Body*, and the *Choroid*. It contains 2 sets of muscles with opposing actions, which allow the size of the *Pupil* to be adjusted under neural control. Only the innermost layer of the eye, the *Retina*, contains neurons that are sensitive to light and can transmit visual signals to the *Optical Nerve*. The *Macula* is a part of the *Retina* responsible for the central vision (sharp, clear, fine detail, straight-ahead vision). The *Macula* has a very high concentration of photoreceptor cells. (*B*) The interaction of electromagnetic radiation to human eye tissues. The optical hazards are associated with the frequency and penetration of the different electromagnetic radiations. Ozone is a gas present in the upper layers of the atmosphere and serves as an exogenous protection layer against harmful ultraviolet (UV) radiation. UV can cause photochemical injury to the cornea (photokeratitis) and lens (cataract) of the eye (180–400 nm). Thermal injury to the retina of the eye is like to happen from 400 to 1400 nm; blue-light photochemical can injure the retina of the eye (principally 400–550 nm); near-infrared thermal hazards to the lens (approximately 800–3000 nm); thermal injury (burns) of the cornea of the eye (approximately 1400 nm to 1 mm); thermal or photochemical injury to the skin from high irradiances.

anatomy. Different investigations have shown that exposure to light of specific wavelengths or intensity may induce severe damage to the eye.[15,16] This type of damage is called light-induced damage. The eyes are at risk of injury from acute and long-term exposure to solar and artificial optical radiation (**Fig. 2**B). The severe dangers that UV radiation presents to both eyes and skin are well established. Increasing evidence has alerted scientists and clinicians to the damage that long-term exposure to visible light may cause to retinal photoreceptors.

Light can cause damage via 3 mechanisms: photomechanical, photothermal, and photochemical.[6] Photomechanical damage is due to a rapid increase in the amount of energy captured by the retinal pigment epithelium (RPE), which may cause irreversible damage to the RPE and lead to photoreceptor damage. This type of retinal damage depends on the amount of energy absorbed and not on the spectral composition of the light. Photothermal damage occurs when the retina and the RPE are exposed to brief (<10 s) but intense light that significantly increases the temperature of these tissues. These injuries can happen to patients and dental personnel who do not wear appropriate personal protective equipment (PPE).[17] They are primarily caused via accidental direct exposure to high-power light irradiation from imprudent use of LCUs by an untrained operator. These accidents can be very severe with lasers, as they can sustain the high power over longer distances due to the coherence of the light beam. When using a dental LCU, the major concern is that cumulative irradiation of the eye may cause permanent damage to the macula and the RPE over the long term.

A more common type of retinal damage is photochemical damage, which occurs when the eyes are exposed to high-intensity light in the visible range (390–600 nm).[6] Several lines of evidence suggest that visual photopigments (eg, rhodopsin and cone opsins) are involved in this type of damage. Early studies also provided evidence that the action spectrum for light-induced photoreceptor damage is similar to the absorption spectrum of rhodopsin. Still, later studies indicated that blue light (400–440 nm) might be more damaging; this has been termed the "blue-light hazard."[18] **Fig. 3** shows the blue-light hazard function defined as the capability of light to produce photochemical retinal damage as a function of wavelength. Current studies suggest that there are 2 distinct types of photochemical damage. The first type is associated with short but intense exposure to light affecting the RPE. The second type is associated with more prolonged but less intense light exposure, affecting the outer segment of the photoreceptors. Short (up to 12 hours) exposure to blue light may induce damage in the RPE (in primates),[19] and a clear relationship has been found between the extent of the damage and the oxygen concentration.[20] Because antioxidative physiologic processes (ie, lipofuscin mediation) can reduce the harm associated with oxidative processes, it is recommended that the radiance, weighted by the blue-light hazard function, received by the eye should not exceed an average of 10 mW/(cm^2−sr) over a total viewing time of up to 167 minutes in a day.

Because the peak absorption for CQ is about 455 to 481 nm, dental LCUs are optimized to perform in the wavelength range where the blue-light retinal injury also occurs. A previous study[13] demonstrated that under clinically relevant conditions, at a viewing distance of 40 cm, the daily maximum permissible cumulative exposure time to blue light from the LCU is 7 seconds (5 mW/cm^2) and approximately 11 minutes (630–690 seconds) (0.053 mW/cm^2) for direct and indirect, reflected light, respectively. When wearing loupes, there is an increase in the radiant flux (mW) entering

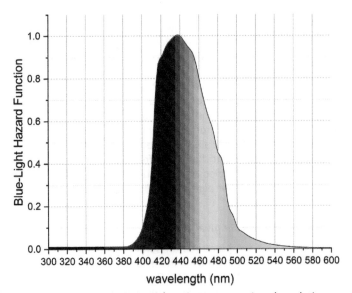

Fig. 3. Spectrum of the blue-light hazard function representing the relative spectral sensitivity of the human eye to the visible light. It is based on the relative spectral effectiveness of optical radiation to induce retinal photochemical injury. The blue-light retinal injury occurs primarily from exposure in the wavelength range between 380 and 550 nm, with the sensitivity of the retina peaking at approximately 440 nm.

the eye. Although the radiant flux received by the eye is greater when loupes are used, the image is magnified and therefore distributed over a broader area of the retina, causing the calculated maximum cumulative daily exposure time to increase to between 16 and 28 minutes. Even so, this maximum daily exposure may be easily exceeded by dentists who place more than 10 restorations a day or by orthodontists or their assistants when bonding brackets onto teeth. Also, the beneficial effect of eye movements to reduce the time-averaged retinal irradiance for a small source may be reduced because loupes induce a greater fixation of looking at one spot on a tooth.

The second type of light-induced photochemical damage occurs with more prolonged (12–48 hours) but less intense light exposure.[6] Several publications suggest that long-term chronic exposure to blue light may accelerate retinal aging and age-related macular degeneration.[15] This type of damage was initially observed in albino rats and other species. The cones seem to be more vulnerable compared with the rods. Although neural retina in humans and rodents have differences in organization and sensitivity to light, the RPE is highly analogous. It has the same functions and ages in the same way in most species. Therefore, phototoxicity data from animal models concerning RPE should be more closely related to human phototoxicity. It is important to note that the methods used to calculate those values were the same for primates and rodents. Recent studies have shown that radiant exposure of 0.5 J/cm^2 already causes cell death, and if the blue-light hazard weighting is considered, this global dose corresponds to 0.06 J/cm^2; this means that cell death with a dose of blue light about 180-fold smaller than the exposure limit values is being detected in animal studies. This evidence suggests that the phototoxicity data obtained in primates and used to establish the current regulations related to the photobiological safety of light sources must also be reevaluated.

Intrinsically photosensitive retinal ganglion cells control body temperature, hormonal levels, sleep duration and quality, cognitive performance, and other physiologic variables.[6] However, excessive exposure to blue light can also disrupt the circadian cycles causing fatigue, stress, mood disorders, and other physiologic and psychological issues. Chronic light exposure at the wrong time, at night during shift work, for example, may contribute to shifts of the circadian clock phase, dependent on duration, wavelength, and intensity of light.

Still, the evidence of the detrimental effect of blue light on the retina should be taken with caution. Most of the damaging effects of blue light are demonstrated in animals or isolated cell cultures directly exposed to blue light. In humans, direct evidence of acute light–induced retina damage from accidental high-intensity artificial or sunlight exposure is obvious. However, there is an increased need for observational studies into whether long-term exposure to blue light from LCUs in dental settings causes damage to the retina. Further studies on the ocular hazards of using loupes and the overall cumulative effects of other high-output light sources in the dental office are required.

Potential Hazards to Pulp and Gingival Tissues

Adverse effects of elevated temperatures on dentin and pulpal structures are significant. According to the most-cited study in the field, as temperature increased (higher than normal oral temperature) from 5.5 to 11°C, at 1 mm into dentin, the possibility of pulp necrosis increased from 15% to 60%.[21] However, it is well known that this all depends on the duration and exact nature of the thermal challenge. A follow-up study indicated that an 11.2°C increase would still be considered safe and not damage pulpal tissues.[22] Some in vivo and in vitro measurements have also demonstrated slower temperature changes within the pulp due to dynamic temperature regulation by the surrounding soft tissue and constant blood flow. The temperatures developed at 1 mm into dentin could have been less in a more clinically simulative environment.

These controversial results are attributable to the fact that it is impossible to track the temperature changes in specific localized pulp areas or to precisely determine how much irradiation to these areas is caused by the exposure (**Fig. 4**). Overall, the heat seems not to be the major injury factor, at least in the short term. However, it is certain to play a role in postoperative inflammation or necrosis in the long term, especially when combined with other factors such as caries and high-speed bur injuries.

On the other hand, the blue light also directly irradiates surrounding soft tissues, especially in cervical restorations, crown cementations, or bleaching procedures. This direct irradiation causes a significant reduction in the proliferative activity of the fibroblasts and increases intracellular reactive oxygen species (ROS) levels and mitochondrial disorders regardless of temperature increase.[23]

Mitochondria contain flavin proteins that underlie photoinduced hydrogen peroxide production (**Fig. 5**). All molecules have an excitation wavelength, and ROS are always produced when oxygen is present. In this case, flavins have an excitation wavelength within the blue-light region. Blue light also can release nitric oxide from intracellular stores in mitochondria and contribute to energy depletion and cell death.[24] Gingival recession can be induced by the inhibition of fibroblasts proliferation and the degradation of collagen synthesis due to ROS.

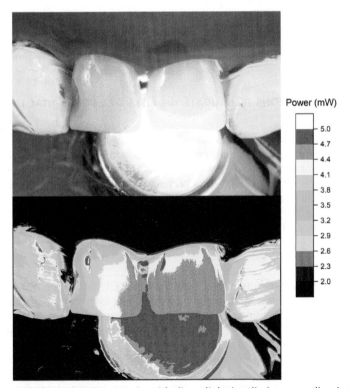

Power (mW)

5.0
4.7
4.4
4.1
3.8
3.5
3.2
2.9
2.6
2.3
2.0

Fig. 4. Class IV light-activation scenario with direct light irradiation spreading intensity according to the origin of exposure. The power estimation was done by image pixel intensity calibration based on previous studies.[13]

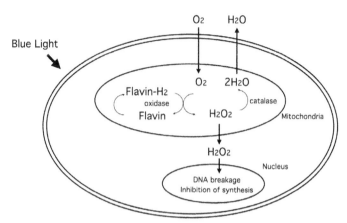

Fig. 5. Photo-induced hydrogen peroxide production in the mitochondria.

Moreover, when these curing lights generate heat, they have the potential to cause damage to the soft tissue. For that reason, the use of high-power LEDs or lasers imposes even more risk of burns. Heat can cause burns because direct heat exposure to cells causes protein denaturation, cell membrane leakage, activation of cytokines, and cessation of blood flow leading to cell death.[25] Depending on the amount of heat, the damage can be immediate or long term.

Thermal injuries occur when energy is transferred from the heat source to the human tissue, causing an increase in the local temperature. When the temperature increases greater than a certain threshold, known to start at 44°C, irreversible cell injury occurs within 6 hours. When the temperature increases beyond 51°C, the injuries are immediate.[26,27]

CLINICAL CONSIDERATIONS TO MITIGATE THE RISKS OF USING DENTAL LIGHT-CURING UNITS

For a health care provider, safety is essential, and as with any other powerful medical device, such as radiography, computed tomography, and MRI, with the proper precautions and training, the benefits of powerful LCUs can outweigh the risks. Despite scientific evidence for visible light risks primarily based on animal studies, sufficient evidence indicates that appropriate precautions should be used by dental personnel when using LCUs.[13,28–31] The American Dental Association Council on Dental Materials, Instruments, and Equipment recommend using protective eyewear when using all LCUs.[32]

Eyewear Protection

Dental personnel should protect their eyes from the LCU to prevent ocular damage. The protective light filters should not completely block longer wavelengths, allowing the visualization of the treatment field while curing adequately. The dentist is responsible for providing appropriate PPE to the patient to prevent potential injuries or side effects caused by medical and dental devices.

The FDA considers curing lights to be Class II medical devices (capable of posing a moderate risk to the patient, user, or both) that must meet approval standards before they can be sold in the United States. Although there are standards for protective eyewear, PPEs purchased aftermarket are Class 1 medical devices (low risk to the patient, user, or both) exempt and not required to submit proof of efficacy and safety before being sold in the United States. LCUs emit light in different wavelength ranges. There is a lack of aftermarket regulation of light protective filters. Not all protective filters are efficient at blocking the shorter wavelengths or longer wavelengths; but even in the worst-case scenario, the filters still have been shown to block more than 97% of the light from the LCU.[33] However, some shields might not filter all the light spectrum appropriately or can be damaged after multiple exposures. Dental professionals need to ensure that the protective glasses' wavelength range as declared by the manufacturer is adequate for the intended function (**Fig. 6**).

Importantly, lasers used for dental light-curing are considered high-powered (>500 mW) Class 4 lasers. A Class 4 laser can cause a significant eye injury if the direct or reflected beam enters the eye. It can burn skin, gingival tissues, and materials, particularly dark and lightweight materials (ie, Rubber Dam). They should be used with extreme caution, and to prevent eye exposure, the operator should always be aware of the beam location. The dentist, the patient, and anyone else in the room should always wear the appropriate laser-certified protective goggles. The laser should not be activated until it is in the patient's mouth over the area to be cured. Also, some PPEs might filter the wavelength, but after consecutive exposures, thermal damage to the plastic shield is expected, as these PPEs do not have resistance to the heat generated by the filtering of high energy. For example, after 3 direct exposures with a Class 4 dental light-curing laser, a regular orange goggle can have its shield's integrity compromised (**Fig. 7**). Although this article is intended for the reader's educational, instructional, and informational purposes, it is not a substitute for a knowledgeable and trained LSO with the duties and responsibilities defined in the ANSI Z136.

Dental personnel have different options for PPEs. Based on previous studies, each one of the PPEs has advantages and disadvantages according to its protective efficacy and convenience (**Fig. 8**).[7] In general, untrained dental personnel believe that the "look away" method is the most convenient and efficient method to avoid blue-light exposure. However, this method is not indicated because the user can no longer monitor the location of the light tip when they look away, and it may result in soft tissue burns, inadequate light curing, and deficient restorations.

	SINGLE-PEAK	MULTI-PEAK	QUADWAVE	LASER
ORANGE GOGGLES	✓ Efficiency 99.5 %	✓ Efficiency 99.2 %	✗ Efficiency 75.0 %	✗ Efficiency 99.7 % ✢ THERMAL DAMAGE
LASER CERTIFIED ORANGE GOGGLES	✓ Efficiency 99.4 %	✓ Efficiency 99.5 %	✗ Efficiency 74.3 %	✓ Efficiency 99.6 %
GREEN GOGGLES	✓ Efficiency 98.1 %	✓ Efficiency 98.3 %	✓ Efficiency 94.9 %	✗ Efficiency 98.0 % ✢ THERMAL DAMAGE

*Data obtained by calculating the relative light transmission (in, %) through the different goggles using each one of the LCUs types. The MARC LC spectrophotometer was used to obtain the data. Single-Peak (Smartlite Pro Cure); Multi-Peak (Valo Grand); Quadwave (Pinkwave); Laser (Monet).
✢ Thermal Damage to the goggle was found after the first exposure and it compromised the shield integrity.

Fig. 6. Eye protection for single peak, multipeak, Quadwave, and laser LCUs.

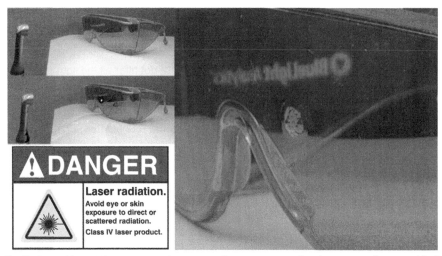

Fig. 7. Dental laser LCU can cause damage to the orange goggles that are not laser certified. The sign of laser radiation hazard for Class IV lasers needs to be visible to patients and dental personnel when using lasers.

Prevention of Pulpal and Gingival Tissue Injuries

Gingival tissue injuries are most likely to happen near the cervical area of the tooth (ie, cervical restorations, crown cementation, bleaching blockers around the gum line, and so forth). In these clinical scenarios, preventing such injuries is performed by carefully positioning the LCU toward the tooth and avoiding exposure to the gingiva. It is known that the curing light should always be positioned parallel to the surface to be light-cured.[3] The axial contour of all facial and buccal surfaces of the teeth are not straight but rather slightly convex. Thus, aiming the curing light appropriately will allow correct exposure to the material being light-cured and reduce the amount of exposure to the surrounding soft tissues (**Fig. 9**).

	ADVANTAGES	DISADVANTAGES
GOGGLES	• Provide optimum protection, eliminate scatter irradiation • Allows for hands-free eye protection	• If using loupes, may be inconvenient to change between the application of dental materials and light curing
LOUPES' INSERTS	• Provide optimum protection, eliminate scatter irradiation • Allows for hands-free eye protection	• Requires more time to properly disinfect between patients.
PADDLES	• May provide adequate coverage for both the dentist and assistant (depending on design and placement of paddle) • Curved paddles allow for better fit around the patient's face than a rectangular paddle	• Requires an extra hand to hold the paddle in place. Does not allow hands-free protection
SHIELDS ATTACHED TO THE LCU	• Can be adjusted to provide best eye protection for the operator	• The surface area of the protective eye filter of most LCUs is not sufficient to protect the dentist and the assistant at the same time • May restrict correct access of the light the restoration
ANTIGLARE CONES	• Easy to use • Allows Hands free protection	• May obstruct the view and may prevent ideal placement of the light tip over the restoration • Can increase the distance between the tooth and the light tip • May not provide sufficient eye protection

Fig. 8. Advantages and disadvantages of different eyewear personal protective equipments.

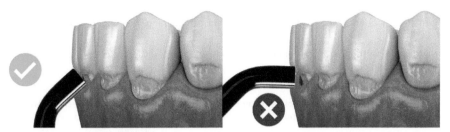

Fig. 9. Left side shows the correct LCU positioning to prevent soft tissue injuries. The tip needs to be in close contact with the restoration, and it should avoid overlap the soft tissues. Right side shows the tip inclined toward the gingival tissue.

Interestingly, rubber dam isolation cannot protect gingiva when high radiant exposure values are delivered. The presence of a rubber dam does not entirely block the light and instead increases the probability of gingival burns because of the rubber dam's heat absorption.[34]

For that reason, it is also thoughtful to prevent the overheating induced by the light-curing process. The most efficient way to overcome this problem is to directly blow air from an air syringe on the tooth that is being light-cured.[35] The air will cool down the tooth and avoid temperature increase. Of course, while light curing, the dentist needs both hands to hold the curing light and stabilize it on the tooth surface being light-cured. Thus, training dental assistants to hold safety orange blockers and blow air on the tooth being cured can be very handy to maintain safety and efficiency.

The cooling down method using the air syringe does not only protect the gingiva from burn injuries but prevents possible overheating of the pulp tissue while light-curing deep restorations. Although the heat seems not to be the major factor of injury in the short term, it can cause postoperative inflammation and induce necrosis of the pulp in the long term and should not be disregarded.[36]

SUMMARY

LCUs are extensively used in dentistry to polymerize dental materials. These materials require high-powered blue light (from 420 to 495 nm) to be efficiently cured in a short curing time. However, cumulative exposure to intense blue light is associated with severe ocular pathologies such as retinal damage and potentially macular degeneration. Also, LCUs pose risks of injuries to the patients' skin, gingival, and pulpal tissues. Nevertheless, the use of high-powered LCUs by trained dental personnel with appropriate safety measures can mitigate the risks and provide patients efficient, high-quality dental care offered by materials with adequate photopolymerization.

CLINICS CARE POINTS

- LCUs used should be approved medical devices, and the eye protection must meet photobiological safety standards.

- It is recommended to use the PPEs provided by the manufacturer of the LCU. However, if a third-party manufactures the orange shields or glasses, ensure that they protect against the wavelengths emitted by the LCU in use.

- If using lasers, make sure to train your dental personnel. Use the laser in a safe, close environment; display the laser radiation sign and be cautious of the use of high-power LCUs.

- To avoid accidents, wear appropriate PPE when manipulating, cleaning, or using a dental LCU.
- Do not leave the LCU in the high-power mode and remove the batteries, if possible, for cleaning and disinfection.
- Never direct the tip of the LCUs directly onto skin and gingival tissues.
- Avoid pulpal inflammation by blowing air on the tooth while light-curing the restorations in close proximity to the dental pulp.

DISCLOSURE

The authors have no commercial or financial conflicts of interest with this article.

REFERENCES

1. Fouassier JP, Lalevée J. Photoinitiators for polymer synthesis: scope, reactivity, and efficiency. Wiley; 2013.
2. Leprince JG, Palin WM, Hadis MA, et al. Progress in dimethacrylate-based dental composite technology and curing efficiency. Dent Mater 2013;29(2): 139–56.
3. Price RB, Ferracane JL, Shortall AC. Light-curing units: a review of what we need to know. J Dent Res 2015;94(9):1179–86.
4. Rueggeberg FA. State-of-the-art: dental photocuring–a review. Dent Mater 2011; 27(1):39–52.
5. Bayne SC, Ferracane JL, Marshall GW, et al. The evolution of dental materials over the past century: silver and gold to tooth color and beyond. J Dent Res 2019;98(3):257–65.
6. Tosini G, Ferguson I, Tsubota K. Effects of blue light on the circadian system and eye physiology. Mol Vis 2016;22:61–72.
7. Fluent MT, Ferracane JL, Mace JG, et al. Shedding light on a potential hazard: dental light-curing units. J Am Dent Assoc 2019;150(12):1051–8.
8. Bruzell Roll EM, Jacobsen N, Hensten-Pettersen A. Health hazards associated with curing light in the dental clinic. Clin Oral Investig 2004; 8(3):113–7.
9. Ecodesign and energy labelling for lighting products: government response. European Union; 2009. IP/08/1909.
10. Jandt KD, Mills RW. A brief history of LED photopolymerization. Dent Mater 2013; 29(6):605–17.
11. de Oliveira DC, Rocha MG, Gatti A, et al. Effect of different photoinitiators and reducing agents on cure efficiency and color stability of resin-based composites using different LED wavelengths. J Dent 2015;43(12):1565–72.
12. Moszner N, Fischer UK, Ganster B, et al. Benzoyl germanium derivatives as novel visible light photoinitiators for dental materials. Dent Mater 2008;24(7): 901–7.
13. Price RB, Labrie D, Bruzell EM, et al. The dental curing light: a potential health risk. J Occup Environ Hyg 2016;13(8):639–46.
14. Reis AF, Vestphal M, Amaral RCD, et al. Efficiency of polymerization of bulk-fill composite resins: a systematic review. Braz Oral Res 2017;31(suppl 1):e59.
15. Wenzel A, Grimm C, Samardzija M, et al. Molecular mechanisms of light-induced photoreceptor apoptosis and neuroprotection for retinal degeneration. Prog Retin Eye Res 2005;24(2):275–306.

16. Organisciak DT, Vaughan DK. Retinal light damage: mechanisms and protection. Prog Retin Eye Res 2010;29(2):113–34.

17. Stamatacos C, Harrison JL. The possible ocular hazards of LED dental illumination applications. J Tenn Dent Assoc 2013;93(2):25–9 [quiz: 30-21].

18. Guidelines on limits of exposure to broad-band incoherent optical radiation (0.38 to 3 microM). International Commission on Non-Ionizing Radiation Protection. Health Phys 1997;73(3):539–54.

19. Ham WT Jr, Ruffolo JJ Jr, Mueller HA, et al. Histologic analysis of photochemical lesions produced in rhesus retina by short-wave-length light. Invest Ophthalmol Vis Sci 1978;17(10):1029–35.

20. Ruffolo JJ Jr, Ham WT Jr, Mueller HA, et al. Photochemical lesions in the primate retina under conditions of elevated blood oxygen. Invest Ophthalmol Vis Sci 1984;25(8):893–8.

21. Zach L, Cohen G. Pulp response to externally applied heat. Oral Surg Oral Med Oral Pathol 1965;19:515–30.

22. Baldissara P, Catapano S, Scotti R. Clinical and histological evaluation of thermal injury thresholds in human teeth: a preliminary study. J Oral Rehabil 1997;24(11):791–801.

23. Yoshida A, Yoshino F, Makita T, et al. Reactive oxygen species production in mitochondria of human gingival fibroblast induced by blue light irradiation. J Photochem Photobiol B 2013;129:1–5.

24. Hockberger PE, Skimina TA, Centonze VE, et al. Activation of flavin-containing oxidases underlies light-induced production of H2O2 in mammalian cells. Proc Natl Acad Sci U S A 1999;96(11):6255–60.

25. Purschke M, Laubach HJ, Anderson RR, et al. Thermal injury causes DNA damage and lethality in unheated surrounding cells: active thermal bystander effect. J Invest Dermatol 2010;130(1):86–92.

26. Henriques FC, Moritz AR. Studies of thermal injury: I. the conduction of heat to and through skin and the temperatures attained therein. A theoretical and an experimental investigation. Am J Pathol 1947;23(4):530–49.

27. Payne-James J. Encyclopedia of forensic and legal medicine. Amsterdam: Elsevier, Acad. Press; 2005.

28. Ahmed AG, Raziq AH. Evaluation of light-emitting diodes' effects on the expression level of P53 and EGFR in the gingival tissues of albino rats. Medicina (Kaunas) 2019;55(9):605.

29. Yoshino F, Yoshida A. Effects of blue-light irradiation during dental treatment. Jpn Dent Sci Rev 2018;54(4):160–8.

30. Price RBT. Light curing in dentistry. Dent Clin North Am 2017;61(4):751–78.

31. Labrie D, Moe J, Price RB, et al. Evaluation of ocular hazards from 4 types of curing lights. Journal 2011;77:b116.

32. The effects of blue light on the retina and the use of protective filtering glasses. Council on dental materials, instruments, and equipment. J Am Dent Assoc 1986;112(4):533–5.

33. Soares CJ, Rodrigues MP, Vilela AB, et al. Evaluation of eye protection filters used with broad-spectrum and conventional LED curing lights. Braz Dent J 2017;28(1):9–15.

34. Maucoski C, Zarpellon DC, Dos Santos FA, et al. Analysis of temperature increase in swine gingiva after exposure to a Polywave((R)) LED light curing unit. Dent Mater 2017;33(11):1266–73.

35. Zarpellon DC, Runnacles P, Maucoski C, et al. Controlling in vivo, human pulp temperature rise caused by LED curing light exposure. Oper Dent 2019;44(3): 235–41.

36. Gross DJ, Dávila-Sánchez A, Runnacles P, et al. In vivo temperature rise and acute inflammatory response in anesthetized human pulp tissue of premolars having class V preparations after exposure to Polywave® LED light curing units. Dent Mater 2020;36(9):1201–13.

Bioactive Restorative Dental Materials—The New Frontier

Mary Anne S. Melo, DDS, PhD[a,b,*], Lamia Mokeem, DDS, MS[a], Jirun Sun, MS, PhD[c]

KEYWORDS

- Antibacterial • Bioactive materials • Dental caries • Oral biofilms • Resin composites

KEY POINTS

- This review presents recent advances and the current state-of-the-art of bioactive materials for dental restorations.
- The current effort has been directed toward developing dental materials that can inhibit biofilms and prevent tooth mineral loss.
- Various resin compositions combined with a wide range of synthetic polymers and nanoparticles have been evaluated to impart bioactivity.
- The developing bioactive materials were subjected to simulated clinical conditions ranging from mechanically loaded testing, assessments against pathogenic clinical isolates, and artificial aging, all with highly favorable outcomes.
- An additional possibility includes reducing the shrinkage stress of the resin restoration together with imparting material bioactivity.

INTRODUCTION

The development of bioactive materials for dental resin restorations is a rising field of investigation in dentistry, providing inspiring ideas to build novel preventive and treatment strategies for reducing the recurrence of carious lesions around restored teeth.[1] Secondary (or recurrent) caries is termed as "lesions at the margins of existing restorations" or "caries associated with restorations or sealants".[2] Secondary caries lesions are the main late complication of dental restorations, limiting their life span and generating costs by repeated reinterventions.[3] As the first-choice material for direct restoration, resin composites have faced increasing failure rates due to secondary caries, requiring dentists to replace this type of material more often.[4] Globally, the

[a] Program in Dental Biomedical Sciences, University of Maryland School of Dentistry, 650 West Baltimore Street, Baltimore, MD 21201, USA; [b] Division of Operative Dentistry, Department of General Dentistry, University of Maryland Dental School, 650 West Baltimore Street, Baltimore, MD 21201, USA; [c] The Forsyth Institute, Harvard School of Dental Medicine Affiliate, 245 First Street, Cambridge, MA 02142, USA
* Corresponding author. 650 West Baltimore Street, Dental School Building, Room 3201, 3rd floor, Baltimore, MD 21201.
E-mail address: mmelo@umaryland.edu
Twitter: @DrMaryAnneMelo (M.A.S.M.)

Dent Clin N Am 66 (2022) 551–566
https://doi.org/10.1016/j.cden.2022.05.005
0011-8532/22/© 2022 Elsevier Inc. All rights reserved.

replacement of failed restorations represents a heavy burden on health care expenditure, accounting for more than 50% of all operative dentistry.[5] In the United States, replacements for failed restorations are reported to be more than 200 million annually.[6]

Secondary caries is a complex, multifactorial process connecting the etiologic factors of primary caries with the specific characteristics of the restorative material involved. Secondary caries located at the gingival margin of class II and V composite restorations can often result from gaps between the restoration and the tooth, allowing acidic fluids or cariogenic biofilm to enter the interface (**Fig. 1**). However, the established factors relevant to caries development are required (presence of a cariogenic biofilm, continuous supply of fermentable carbohydrates, and imbalance in mineral loss).[7,8] In addition, composites also seem to encourage the growth of cariogenic bacteria on their surface, which has been associated with specific surface properties, the release of components, and lack of antibacterial properties.[9]

Therefore, over the last decade, the clinical data have pushed the development of new dental restorative materials to reduce rates of secondary caries around resin composite restorations.[3] The possibility that restorative materials could have bioactive properties has created excitement among dentists as an opportunity to provide better preventive functionally esthetic restorations to their patients. Based on this, the search for strategies to impart bioactivity to resin materials has grown tremendously.

Accompanying this exploratory journey into the development of bioactive materials for dental restorations is uncertainty about the best or proper terminology to be used when describing these materials. In an American Dental Association News publication from June 2018,[10] the term "biointeractive" was considered. The definition of biointeractive refers to the ability to release ions, including those present in tooth minerals, which is a property associated with being "biointeractive." Ions released from a "biointeractive" restorative material or cement may enter saliva, driving the process of remineralization in the surrounding tooth structure. The definition was also discussed during the 2018 Northern Lights consensus conference held in Oslo, Norway.[11] It was

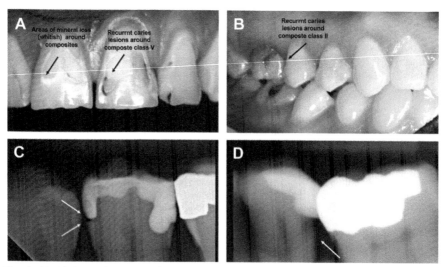

Fig. 1. (*A, B*) Secondary caries located around class V and II composite restorations. (*C*) Radiographic image shows a large gap between the tooth and restoration. (*D*) Radiographic image displays a secondary caries lesion underneath proximal composite restoration. The yellow arrows show the presence of gaps between the tooth and restoration.

suggested that dental restorative materials may be called "bioactive" if, in addition to their primary function of restoring or replacing missing tooth structure, they can actively stimulate or direct specific cellular and/or tissue responses or control interactions with microbiological species.[11] To date, no universally agreed-on definitive definition of bioactivity exists in dentistry, and this may lead to confusion or at least inconsistency. Therefore, it is important to clarify one's meaning when discussing bioactivity for dental restoratives.

Considering resin-based materials, where the intended positive outcome is to reduce the occurrence of secondary caries, the term bioactivity can be applied when the bioactive agent can reduce dysbiosis by reducing disease-promoting bacteria or avoiding the chemical imbalance that leads to tooth mineral loss.[12] **Fig. 2** indicates the routes of bioactivity toward dental caries prevention via dental restorative materials: route 1—the release or contact with bioactive additives that can modulate or suppress bacterial metabolism, inevitably reducing biofilm growth, and route 2—the release of relevant ions, such as calcium ions, to promote remineralization. Focusing on the anticaries behavior of bioactive materials, this review discusses the advancements made during the last 5 years in anticaries strategies based on bioactive additives/compounds used with other classes of materials. As resin composites comprise 2 constituents, one being organic and functioning as the matrix phase and the other being inorganic and serving as the reinforcing phase, these constituents are the primary targets for modifications. As a result, various compositions of dental resins have been combined with synthetic polymers using a diverse range of fabrication methods.

FORMULATING BIOACTIVE RESTORATIVE MATERIALS

Developing resin-based dental materials for restorations (dental adhesives, resin composites, luting agent additives, and sealants, among others) must satisfactorily meet the core properties required for their clinical application.[13] In addition, any strategies and technologies to impart bioactivity require novel dental materials to meet the basic

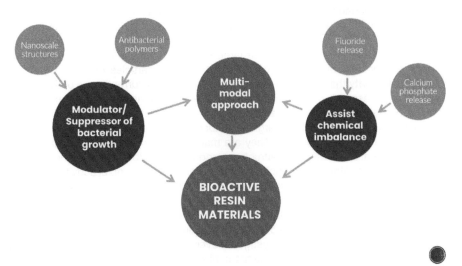

Fig. 2. Routes of bioactivity preventing dental caries using dental restorative materials: route 1—using bioactive additives to modulate or suppress bacterial metabolism, inevitably reducing biofilm growth and route 2—ion release to enhance remineralization.

properties of their nonbioactive counterpart materials. For example, resin-based sealants must possess a high degree of wettability, flow, and viscosity that allow the penetration into the occlusal fissures and grooves of the teeth. Other core properties are the resistance to abrasion and fracture, degree of conversion, and bond strength.[14]

The manner in which the dental polymers and the bioactive additives are combined to produce a final bioactive formulation is obviously very important, and the distribution of components within the resin formulation can be critical to the desired functionality. For example, poor degree of conversion of dental resin monomers, elution of unpolymerized monomers, and degradation of polymeric chains by enzymatic and hydrolytic challenges are drawbacks currently faced by dental polymers.[15] Achieving a uniform composition throughout the mixture is critical, as incorporating bioactive additives into the resin frequently decreases the core properties or the bioactivity profile if they are not well distributed.[1] The choice of the type of bioactive agent and ratio between the resin and inorganic fillers participating in such combinations can greatly affect the resulting bulk physical and mechanical properties of the intended bioactive restorative materials. In addition, the bioactivity properties can be adjusted by tuning the composite composition, including both the polymeric networks[16] and the reinforcing fillers. For example, for bioactive glass nanoparticles, the rate of ion release is determined by the Ca:P ratio, composition, and microstructure.[17] Based on that, many ongoing research studies focus on finding a suitable combination of mechanical/physicochemical properties and bioactivity profiles. However, the most desirable bioactive profiling should not be a priority at the cost of the physical or mechanical properties required for the materials' functionality, else clinical outcomes will be poor.

Bioactive Additives to Modulate/Suppress Bacterial Growth

Materials science studies have looked for additives or compounds that can effectively minimize the growth of biofilms on restorative materials.[16] Strategies include incorporating inorganic and organic additives.

Nanosized antibacterial structures

The fabrication of nanosized antibacterial structures achieved via different nanotechnologies has increasingly been used to develop bioactive materials.[18] In terms of antibacterial applications, both multifunctional nanoengineered materials and nonnanoengineered structures with very their large surface-to-volume ratio have a unique advantage over their bulk counterparts.[19] Metallic nanoparticles displayed greater antibacterial activity than traditional macro metals, which is currently one of the focus areas in dental research.[20] Moreover, nanoengineered materials are good candidates for incorporation into resin matrices due to their inorganic nature, unique physiochemical properties, and multimode synergistic antibacterial performance, offering multiple pathways to inactivate bacteria.[21] They are mainly metal and metal oxide nanoparticles but also carbon-based nanostructures and quantum dots, among others.[22]

Metal and metal oxide nanoparticles pose substantial antimicrobial activity by metal ion release, oxidative stress induction, and nonoxidative mechanisms.[23] Silver, zinc, titanium, copper, and magnesium ions have been used to develop metal and metal oxide nanoparticles.[24] The antibacterial effect of the resin materials (bonding adhesives and composites) containing these constituents, mainly silver and zinc and oxide nanostructures, has been extensively investigated over the years. The materials containing these metals have shown activity against a wide range of oral bacterial pathogens, including *Streptococcus mutans*, that are strongly associated with the caries process.[25] Recently, Garcia and coworkers formulated a dental resin with 7.5 wt% zinc oxide nanoparticles showing a substantial bacterial reduction of saliva-derived biofilm, as described in **Fig. 3**.[25] The drawbacks of this strategy are uncontrollable release with limited antibacterial activity following an initial burst of release, lack of long-term efficacy against bacterial growth, and nanoparticles that are prone to agglomeration due to their high surface area.[26]

Recently, a new perspective on metal oxide additives was investigated.[27] The smallest particles of zinc and tantalum oxides that could be incorporated into restorative materials were synthesized. These quantum dots have been tested in resins to overcome the typical agglomeration of nanoparticles.[28] Different from classic

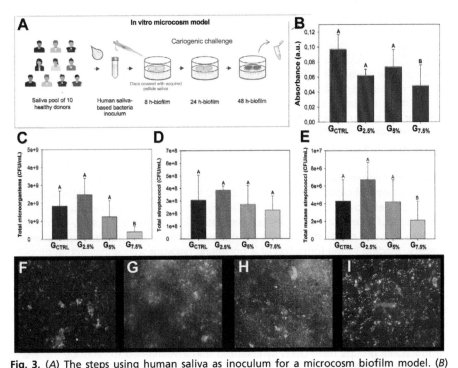

Fig. 3. (A) The steps using human saliva as inoculum for a microcosm biofilm model. (B) Metabolic activity for the following groups: control group—no zinc oxide particles incorporated (GCTRL), zinc oxide particles at 2.5 wt% group (G2.5%), zinc oxide particles at 5 wt% group (G5%), and zinc oxide particles at 7.5 wt% group (G7.5%). Adhesives with zinc oxide particles at 7.5 wt% (G7.5%) significantly reduced the metabolic activity of biofilms ($P<.05$). (C–E) CFU counting results for (C) total microorganisms, (D) total streptococci, and (E) mutans streptococci, respectively. There was no difference among groups up to 5 wt.% of ZnO addition for total microorganism viability ($P>.05$). The group with 7.5 wt.% of ZnO showed the lowest value of CFU/mL for total microorganisms ($P<.05$). For the evaluation of total streptococci (3D), there was no difference among groups ($P>.05$). For total mutans, streptococci (E), G7.5% showed lower viability than other groups ($P<.05$). (F–I) Microscopy images of live/dead assay. F represents an image of biofilm grown for the control group—no zinc oxide particles incorporated (GCTRL); G represents an image of biofilm for the group containing zinc oxide particles at 2.5 wt% (G2.5%); H represents an image of biofilm for the group containing zinc oxide particles at 5 wt% (G5%); and I represents an image of biofilm for the group containing zinc oxide particles at 7.5 wt% (G7.5%). More pronounced areas of dead microorganisms represented by orange/yellow color can be seen within the biofilms. Note the absence or minimal presence of denoted orange/yellow color in the images of a control group.

nanoparticles, quantum dots, or "artificial atoms," do not exceed 10 nm in dimension, and, surprisingly, they showed stability in a colloidal system even after 6 months of storage.[27,29,30]

In addition to oxides, polymeric nanoparticles also have been used to impart bioactivity. Polymeric nanoparticles can be loaded with active compounds entrapped within or surface-adsorbed onto the polymeric core. The term "nanoparticle" stands for nanocapsules and nanospheres, distinguished by the morphologic structure. Antimicrobial polymeric nanoparticles are highlighted due to their antibacterial activity and nontoxicity to human cells.[31] In 2018, a study reported that incorporating 5 wt% of a new quaternary ammonium methacryloxy silane, prepared from sol-gel chemistry, into an experimental adhesive formulation achieved concomitant antibacterial and anti-proteolytic effects without compromising dentin bond strength.[32] Following studies focused on this approach used quaternary ammonium silica dioxide (QASi) nanoparticles.[33] QASi particles are synthesized to form a high concentration of antimicrobial groups covalently bound onto a carrier core, such as silica. The resulting micro- or nanosized QASi particles mixed with other fillers led to developing a commercially available resin composite (Nobio Infinix, Nobio Ltd., Kadima, Israel). Last year, an in situ clinical study showed that composites containing QASi particles significantly reduced demineralization in enamel adjacent to a 38-μm gap over 4 weeks compared with a conventional composite.[34]

Antibacterial polymers

In the panorama of bioactive additives designed for dental materials to modulate/suppress bacterial growth, antibacterial quaternary ammonium monomers have perhaps been the most investigated.[35] They possess intrinsic antimicrobial activity within their structure and can copolymerize with the methacrylate monomers commonly used in dentistry, leading to the formation of a polymeric network with antimicrobial properties.[36] The cationic moiety exerts antimicrobial effects by destabilizing the negatively charged cell membrane of microbes.[37] When incorporated into the resin at concentrations of 2.5% to 10%, the resin materials have nonleaching contact-bactericidal effects, low cytotoxicity, and optimal mechanical properties, such as flexural strength and modulus.[36,38] Based on these results, a multitude of synthetic monomers containing different positive quaternary amine charges, alkyl chain lengths, and positions of the functional groups have been synthesized and investigated to produce materials with enhanced antibacterial effect.[39,40] Recently, Ibrahim and colleagues[41] described the anticaries performance of a quaternary ammonium monomer with an alkyl chain length of 16 carbons. Adding 5% dimethylaminohexadecyl methacrylate into a resin imparted a detrimental biological effect on *S mutans* by reducing colony-forming unit counts (CFU) and metabolic activity as measured by exopolysaccharide synthesis. In addition, reduced overall acid production and reduced tolerance to oxygen stress, 2 major virulence factors of this microorganism, were shown. Yu and colleagues[42] observed similar performance with a quaternary ammonium monomer with the same structure but a shorter alkyl chain length (only 12 carbon). Investigations on the role of the alkyl chain length have pointed out major differences in the antibacterial performance. For short-chained quaternary ammonium, the antimicrobial activity relies merely on a positively charged ammonium group coupling with a negatively charged bacterial membrane to disrupt membrane functions, alter the balance of essential ions, interrupt protein activity, and damage bacterial DNA, whereas, for long-chained quaternary ammonium compounds, some have postulated a double-killing effect: (1) the positive charges and (2) the additional antimicrobial activity by insertion of the carbon chain into the bacterial membrane, resulting in physical disruption.[40,43]

Even with a strong and long-lasting antibacterial effect, incorporating these recently developed quaternary ammonium monomers into dental resins has shown some adverse effects. Most of the designed and investigated antibacterial monomers are monomethacrylates with pendant quaternary ammonium moieties. This structure has stability problems due to the hydrolysis of ester functional groups, decreasing physical performance and causing biosafety concerns.[44] To solve these problems, quaternary ammonium monomers have been recently synthesized with 2 or more methacrylate groups.[45,46] Wang and colleagues[45] suggested that a quaternary ammonium salt monomer with 4 polymerizable methacrylate groups can improve the cross-linking density and performance of the dental resin.

Bioactive Additives to Assist Chemical Imbalance at the Interface Tooth/Material

At physiologic conditions, saliva has a chemical balance of calcium (Ca) and phosphate (Pi) in saturated concentrations compared with the tooth mineral content. The influx-efflux of these ions provides a buffering capacity to neutralize the pH generated after acidic encounters in the oral cavity, and saliva acts as a carrier of essential ions, such as fluoride, calcium, and phosphate.[47] At a low pH, saliva is undersaturated with calcium and phosphate ions, and tooth demineralization can occur.[48]

The development of calcium, phosphate, and fluoride ion–releasing materials was based on the premise that the ions released from a "bioactive" restorative material would supersaturate the surrounding microenvironment of the tooth/material interface when under acidic attack. This responsive boost of relevant ions would prevent demineralization and promote remineralization. The ions released also interfere with the growth of cariogenic bacteria by maintaining a neutral/basic environment, consequently inhibiting their proliferation.[49]

Recent reports[50,51] have summarized the current commercially available ion-releasing dental materials. Most of them can be classified as glass ionomer materials based on their formulation, with the recent introduction of materials with greater resin content and reactive fillers (ie, those activated by acids), whose composition varies according to the manufacturer. Therefore, these materials differ somewhat from the first generation of resin-modified glass ionomers.[50] They mostly claimed to release fluoride ions and were introduced to the market in 2013. Examples of the current commercially available ion-releasing dental materials are Activa BioActive Restorative (Pulpdent Corporation, Watertown, MA, USA), Cention N (Ivoclar-Vivadent, AG, Schaan, Liechtenstein), and Surefil One (Dentsply-Sirona, Konstanz, Germany).

Despite being available for clinical use, the behavior of the commercially available ion-releasing dental restorative materials in the short and long term remains unclear. Because of a lack of a substantial number of clinical studies, the evidence necessary to show which materials are and are not effective and have a substantial positive impact on the patient's oral health is not yet available.

Regarding the bioactive materials under investigation, calcium phosphates (CaP) have been explored as sources of calcium and phosphates ions.[52] Over the last 2 decades, CaP fillers, such as hydroxyapatite, amorphous calcium phosphates, nano-calcium phosphates, and mono-, di-, and tetracalcium phosphates have been incorporated into resin materials.[53–55] Amorphous calcium phosphate is the most commonly found CaP phase in studies with experimental dental resins. In particular, when CaP is presented in nanosized particles, the high surface area enables more ion releases using a relatively lower filler level.[56] CaP derivatives have been used as co-fillers in the inorganic content of a variety of resin-based materials, with promising outcomes of reduced mineral loss or remineralization.[54,55,57]

Some challenges to the inclusion of CaP nanoparticles within dental restorative materials are the compromised mechanical properties due to clustering or leaching-out, the early boost of ion release that is not sustained in the long term, and grayish color attributed to the dental resin when at a concentration range of 20 to 30 wt%.[53] In response to these shortcomings, recent reports have described strategies for recharge and rerelease of calcium and fluoride using different resin matrices.[58] The recharge capacity has shown promising results after 6 recharging/rereleasing cycles with continuous fluoride and calcium ion release measurements after 48 days, as described in **Fig. 4**.

MULTIMODAL APPROACH

Loading multiple bioactive additives into resin materials is a potential strategy for targeting cariogenic biofilm growth and the imbalance of mineral loss.[59,60] In recent years, significant advancements toward the multimodal approach have led to the development of dental materials tailored to exhibit antibacterial and remineralizing effects simultaneously or in combination with other additional properties.[61] Many studies show the combinatory antibiofilm and remineralizing effect as anticaries strategies focusing on the balance between bioactivity, mechanical properties, and durability.[41,62,63] Some bioactive additives can generate synergetic effects and enhance the antibacterial potential.[64,65] For instance, Hesaraki and coworkers[64] formulated a resin composite containing fluoride-releasing fillers, for example, synthetic strontium fluoride (SrF2) nanoparticles, and another antibacterial agent, for example, yttria-stabilized zirconia (YSZ) nanoparticles and poly-ε-l-lysin (ε-PL). A synergy between SrF_2 nanoparticles and ε-PL exhibited a better antibacterial activity in colony reduction than the other samples. In addition, the inclusion of YSZ maintained the mechanical performance in achieving higher antibacterial effects.

The combination of inorganic nanoparticles and polymeric materials to impart anticaries effects have also been explored. Balhaddad and colleagues[66] have investigated formulations containing 2 bioactive agents: antibacterial agent, dimethylamino-hexadecyl methacrylate (DMAHDM) at 3 to 5 wt.%, and remineralization agent, nanosized amorphous calcium phosphate (NACP) at 20 wt.%. These agents were incorporated resin network and evaluated in vitro using microcosm biofilms derived from dental plaque collected from active subgingival cervical periodontitis–associated sites. The DMAHDM-NACP composites significantly inhibited the growth of total microorganisms, *Porphyromonas gingivalis*, *Prevotella intermedia/nigrescens*, *Aggregatibacter actinomycetemcomitans*, and *Fusobacterium nucleatum*, by 3- to 5-log. For the colony isolates from control composites, the composition was typically dominated by the genera *Veillonella, Fusobacterium, Streptococcus, Eikenella*, and *Leptotrichia*, whereas *Fusobacterium* and *Veillonella* dominated the DMAHDM-NACP composites. Moreover, the DMAHDM-NACP composites reduced metabolic and polysaccharide production activity by greater than 80% (**Fig. 5**).

Considerable literature in this area has called attention to the performance of pure bioactive glass particles incorporated in dental resins.[67–70] With calcium, phosphate, and fluoride ion release, low cytotoxicity to dental pulp cells, antibacterial activity, and no impairment of the mechanical surface properties of the bioactive composite, this bioactive additive is promising to inhibit the demineralization and bacterial growth.[67,69,71] Other latest strategies have involved doping bioglass nanoparticles with therapeutic ions, such as silver, lithium, zinc, and copper, mainly in an attempt to boost the antibacterial effect of bioglass.[72–74] Yao and coworkers[74] have explored zinc-calcium-fluoride bioglass as a multifunctional bioactive additive for dental

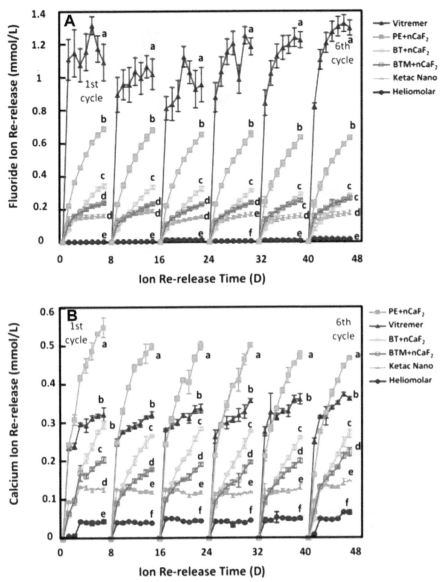

Fig. 4. Following ion exhaustion, nanocomposites with calcium fluoride nanoparticles and commercial material controls were recharged and measured their ion rerelease. (*A*) Fluoride ion recharging cycles and (*B*) calcium ion recharging cycles. In each plot, different letters indicate values that are significantly different from each other at day 7 ($P<.05$).

adhesive. In this study, optimal polymerization conversion resulted in extremely low water sorption and solubility, conceding bond-degradation resistance. In addition, antienzymatic and antibacterial therapeutic effects through gradual ion release from the contained bioactive zinc-calcium-fluoride bioglass were also observed. These properties were obtained while immediate and favorable 1-year aged bond-strength data were found.

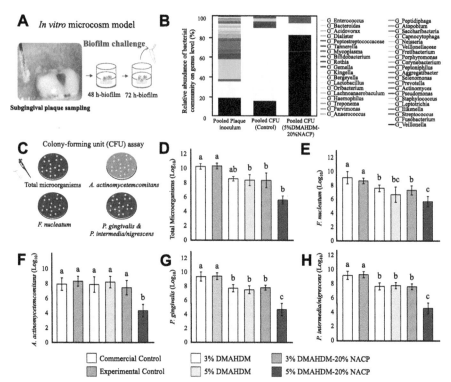

Fig. 5. (*A*) The plaque samples isolated from the subgingival area were used to initiate plaque-derived microcosm biofilms in vitro. (*B*) A color-coded stacked barplot graph shows average bacterial relative abundance on genus level in both groups of pooled plaque inoculum. Pooled plaque inoculum refers to the bacterial composition of the inoculum used to initiate the plaque-derived biofilms. The pooled CFU control refers to the colony-forming unit (CFU) isolates derived from the control composites. The pooled CFU 5%DMAHDM-20%NACP refers to the colony-forming unit (CFU) isolates derived from the biofilm grown over 5%DMAHDM-20%NACP composites. (*C*) The nonselective and selective agar plates used in the CFU assay to count (*D*) total microorganisms, (*E*) Fusobacterium nucleatum, (*F*) Aggregatibacter actinomycetemcomitans, (*G*) Porphyromonas gingivalis, and (*H*) Prevotella intermedia/nigrescens. Values indicated by different letters are statistically different from each other (*P*<.05).

Montoya and colleagues[65] proposed for the first time the use of piezoelectric nanoparticles of barium titanate (BaTiO$_3$) as a multifunctional bioactive filler in dental resin composites, offering combined antibacterial and remineralization effects. In this work, compared with the control, the BaTiO$_3$ composite material showed antibacterial and antibiofilm effects, as evidenced by a substantial reduction in the biofilm biomass, metabolic activity, and numbers of several of the viable bacteria. The best antimicrobial effect was found for lower amounts of BTO (<10%) and small electrical charges (<3.2 pC/cm^2). However, the antibacterial response of this composite can be tuned by varying the filler content and applied mechanical load. Furthermore, the piezoelectric composite showed remineralization capabilities, as evidenced by the formation of calcium phosphate layers with thicknesses ranging from 5 to 23 μm over 7 days for mechanically stimulated composites. The composite's interface with the dentin was subjected to repetitive loading while being submerged in cultures of microorganisms (ie, pathogenic bacteria). After a 6-day biofilm/cyclic loading challenge, the incorporation of piezoelectric fillers in the dental-adhesive composites reduced the bacterial penetration on the bonded interface.

Other multimodal approaches refer to bioactive additives' combined effect with other strategies to improve dental resin stability and durability.[75] Recent studies have moved toward this approach by using a low-shrinkage-stress resin network, for example, a mixture of urethane dimethacrylate (UDMA) and biostable triethylene glycol-divinylbenzene ether (TEGDVBE).[61,76–78] The multifunctional composite containing 3 wt% DMAHDM and 20 wt% NACP, 55.8 wt% of UDMA, and 44.2 wt% of TEGDVBE presented shrinkage stress 36% lower than that of traditional composite control, with similar degrees of conversion of 73.9%. The new composite decreased the biofilm colony-forming units by 4-log orders and substantially reduced biofilm lactic acid production compared with the control composite ($P<.05$). In addition, incorporating DMAHDM into the low-shrinkage-stress composite did not adversely affect the Ca and P ion release.

FUTURE TRENDS

Bioactive dental restorative materials provide a potentially invaluable opportunity to develop additional approaches to fight secondary caries. The available approaches range in complexity, from simple incorporation of bioactive additives to sophisticated and intricate designs to control multiple aspects of caries development around restorations. Each bioactive formulation is tailored to optimize the performance of the intended material, maintaining the core functionality and adding an aspect of bioactivity. These materials have shown the potential to interfere with polymicrobial consortia in vivo and help prevent the recurrence of lesions and maintain the lifespan of restorations. Despite the accomplishments, there are still many challenges to overcome, and most of the investigations are in the early stage of development. Further assessment will be necessary for future clinical translation.

CLINICS CARE POINTS

- Bioactive dental restorative materials provide a potentially invaluable opportunity to develop additional approaches to fight secondary caries.
- Despite the accomplishments, there are still many challenges to overcome, and most of the investigations are in the early stage of development.
- Further assessment will be necessary for future clinical translation.

ACKNOWLEDGMENTS

The study supported by NICDR of the National Institutes of Health under award number R03DE030562. The authors thank Drs Michael Weir, Jack Ferracane, Hockin Xu, Abdulrahman Abu Baker Balhadad, and Isadora Garcia for discussions and experimental help.

DISCLOSURE

The authors have nothing to disclose.

REFERENCES

1. Melo MAS, editor. Designing bioactive polymeric materials for restorative dentistry. London: CRC Press; 2020.
2. Brouwer F, Askar H, Paris S, et al. Detecting Secondary Caries Lesions: A Systematic Review and Meta-analysis. J Dent Res 2016;95(2):143–51.
3. Askar H, Krois J, Göstemeyer G, et al. Secondary caries risk of different adhesive strategies and restorative materials in permanent teeth: Systematic review and network meta-analysis. J Dent 2021;104:103541.
4. Nedeljkovic I, De Munck J, Vanloy A, et al. Secondary caries: prevalence, characteristics, and approach. Clin Oral Investig 2020;24(2):683–91.
5. Eltahlah D, Lynch CD, Chadwick BL, et al. An update on the reasons for placement and replacement of direct restorations. J Dent 2018;72:1–7.
6. Deligeorgi V, Mjör IA, Wilson NH. An overview of reasons for the placement and replacement of restorations. Prim Dent Care J Fac Gen Dent Pract UK 2001; 8(1):5–11.
7. Askar H, Krois J, Göstemeyer G, et al. Secondary caries: what is it, and how it can be controlled, detected, and managed? Clin Oral Investig 2020;24(5):1869–76.
8. Hollanders ACC, Kuper NK, Maske TT, et al. Secondary Caries in situ Models: A Systematic Review. Caries Res 2018;52(6):454–62.
9. Nedeljkovic I, Teughels W, De Munck J, et al. Is secondary caries with composites a material-based problem? Dent Mater 2015;31(11):e247–77.
10. ace_panel_report_bioactive_materials_q2_2018.pdf. Available at: https://www. ada.org/-/media/project/ada-organization/ada/ada-org/files/resources/research/ ace/ace_panel_report_bioactive_materials_q2_2018.pdf?rev=54df56752867427 8a057ca494b0f2539&hash=EEE0910545FF0EF8AEE321EF3698C809. Accessed January 25, 2022.
11. Price RB, Roulet JF. The value of consensus conferences: Peer review by 50 key opinion leaders. Stomatol EDU J 2018;5(4):202–4.
12. Lawson NC, Robles A. Tipping Point: An Update on Curing Lights, Resin Composites, and Matrix Systems. Compend Contin Educ Dent 2017;38(2):120–1.
13. Balhaddad AA, Ibrahim MS, Weir MD, et al. Concentration dependence of quaternary ammonium monomer on the design of high-performance bioactive composite for root caries restorations. Dent Mater Off Publ Acad Dent Mater 2020; 36(8):e266–78.
14. Materials for Direct Restorations. Available at: https://www.ada.org/resources/ research/science-and-research-institute/oral-health-topics/materials-for-direct-restorations. Accessed February 1, 2022.
15. Puoci F. Advanced polymers in medicine. New York: Springer; 2014.
16. Xue J, Wang J, Feng D, et al. Application of Antimicrobial Polymers in the Development of Dental Resin Composite. Molecules 2020;25(20):4738.
17. Ji L, Xu T, Gu J, et al. Preparation of bioactive glass nanoparticles with highly and evenly doped calcium ions by reactive flash nanoprecipitation. J Mater Sci Mater Med 2021;32(5):48.
18. Yougbaré S, Mutalik C, Okoro G, et al. Emerging Trends in Nanomaterials for Antibacterial Applications. Int J Nanomedicine 2021;16:5831–67.
19. Baig N, Kammakakam I, Falath W. Nanomaterials: a review of synthesis methods, properties, recent progress, and challenges. Mater Adv 2021;2(6):1821–71.
20. Balhaddad AA, Garcia IM, Mokeem L, et al. Metal Oxide Nanoparticles and Nanotubes: Ultrasmall Nanostructures to Engineer Antibacterial and Improved Dental Adhesives and Composites. Bioeng Basel Switz 2021;8(10):146.

21. Rawashdeh RY, Sawafta R, Malkawi HI. <p>Dental Materials Incorporated with Nanometals and Their Effect on the Bacterial Growth of Staphylococcus aureus</p>. Int J Nanomedicine 2020;15:4325–31.

22. Monteiro JC, Garcia IM, Leitune VCB, et al. Halloysite nanotubes loaded with alkyl trimethyl ammonium bromide as antibacterial agent for root canal sealers. Dent Mater Off Publ Acad Dent Mater 2019;35(5):789–96.

23. Ghiciuc CM, Ghiciuc ON, Ochiuz L, et al. Antibacterial effects of metal oxides-containing nanomaterials in dentistry. In: 2017 E-Health and Bioengineering Conference (EHB). July 5–9, 2017, Pittsburg, Pennsilvania; 2017:365-368. https://doi.org/10.1109/EHB.2017.7995437.

24. Nizami MZI, Xu VW, Yin IX, et al. Metal and Metal Oxide Nanoparticles in Caries Prevention: A Review. Nanomater Basel Switz 2021;11(12):3446.

25. Garcia IM, Balhaddad AA, Ibrahim MS, et al. Antibacterial response of oral microcosm biofilm to nano-zinc oxide in adhesive resin. Dent Mater Off Publ Acad Dent Mater 2021;37(3):e182–93.

26. Collares FM, Garcia IM, Klein M, et al. Exploring Needle-Like Zinc Oxide Nanostructures for Improving Dental Resin Sealers: Design and Evaluation of Antibacterial, Physical and Chemical Properties. Polymers 2020;12(4):E789.

27. Garcia IM, Souza VS, Scholten JD, et al. Quantum Dots of Tantalum Oxide with an Imidazolium Ionic Liquid as Antibacterial Agent for Adhesive Resin. J Adhes Dent 2020;22(2):207–14.

28. Wrasse EO, Garcia IM, Baierle RJ, et al. Quantum chemistry study of the interaction between ionic liquid-functionalized TiO2 quantum dots and methacrylate resin: Implications for dental materials. Biophys Chem 2020;265:106435.

29. Garcia IM, Souza VS, Hellriegel C, et al. Ionic Liquid-Stabilized Titania Quantum Dots Applied in Adhesive Resin. J Dent Res 2019;98(6):682–8.

30. Garcia IM, Leitune VCB, Visioli F, et al. Influence of zinc oxide quantum dots in the antibacterial activity and cytotoxicity of an experimental adhesive resin. J Dent 2018;73:57–60.

31. Chrószcz M, Barszczewska-Rybarek I. Nanoparticles of Quaternary Ammonium Polyethylenimine Derivatives for Application in Dental Materials. Polymers 2020; 12(11):E2551.

32. Gou YP, Meghil MM, Pucci CR, et al. Optimizing resin-dentin bond stability using a bioactive adhesive with concomitant antibacterial properties and anti-proteolytic activities. Acta Biomater 2018;75:171–82.

33. Zaltsman N, Ionescu AC, Weiss EI, et al. Surface-modified nanoparticles as anti-biofilm filler for dental polymers. PLoS One 2017;12(12):e0189397.

34. Rechmann P, Le CQ, Chaffee BW, et al. Demineralization prevention with a new antibacterial restorative composite containing QASi nanoparticles: an in situ study. Clin Oral Investig 2021;25(9):5293–305.

35. Mitwalli H, Alsahafi R, Balhaddad AA, et al. Emerging Contact-Killing Antibacterial Strategies for Developing Anti-Biofilm Dental Polymeric Restorative Materials. Bioeng Basel Switz 2020;7(3):E83.

36. Garcia IM, Rodrigues SB, de Souza Balbinot G, et al. Quaternary ammonium compound as antimicrobial agent in resin-based sealants. Clin Oral Investig 2020;24(2):777–84.

37. Makvandi P, Jamaledin R, Jabbari M, et al. Antibacterial quaternary ammonium compounds in dental materials: A systematic review. Dent Mater Off Publ Acad Dent Mater 2018;34(6):851–67.

38. Mena Silva PA, Garcia IM, Nunes J, et al. Myristyltrimethylammonium Bromide (MYTAB) as a Cationic Surface Agent to Inhibit Streptococcus mutans Grown over Dental Resins: An In Vitro Study. J Funct Biomater 2020;11(1):E9.

39. Chrószcz MW, Barszczewska-Rybarek IM. Synthesis and Characterization of Novel Quaternary Ammonium Urethane-Dimethacrylate Monomers-A Pilot Study. Int J Mol Sci 2021;22(16):8842.

40. Liang J, Li M, Ren B, et al. The anti-caries effects of dental adhesive resin influenced by the position of functional groups in quaternary ammonium monomers. Dent Mater 2018;34(3):400–11.

41. Ibrahim MS, Ibrahim AS, Balhaddad AA, et al. A Novel Dental Sealant Containing Dimethylaminohexadecyl Methacrylate Suppresses the Cariogenic Pathogenicity of Streptococcus mutans Biofilms. Int J Mol Sci 2019;20(14):E3491.

42. Jinzhao Yu, Huang Xiaoyu, Zhou Xuedong, et al. Anti-caries effect of resin infiltrant modified by quaternary ammonium monomers. J Dent 2020;97:103355.

43. Li F, Weir MD, Xu HHK. Effects of Quaternary Ammonium Chain Length on Antibacterial Bonding Agents. J Dent Res 2013;92(10):932–8.

44. Jaymand M, lotfi M, Abbasian M. Fabrication of novel dental nanocomposites and investigation their physicochemical and biological properties. Mater Res Express 2018;5(3):035406.

45. Wang W, Wu F, Zhang G, et al. Preparation of a highly crosslinked biosafe dental nanocomposite resin with a tetrafunctional methacrylate quaternary ammonium salt monomer. RSC Adv 2019;9(71):41616–27.

46. Fanfoni L, Marsich E, Turco G, et al. Development of di-methacrylate quaternary ammonium monomers with antibacterial activity. Acta Biomater 2021;129:138–47.

47. Naumova EA, Staiger M, Kouji O, et al. Randomized investigation of the bioavailability of fluoride in saliva after administration of sodium fluoride, amine fluoride and fluoride containing bioactive glass dentifrices. BMC Oral Health 2019; 19(1):119.

48. Farooq I, Bugshan A. The role of salivary contents and modern technologies in the remineralization of dental enamel: a narrative review. F1000Research 2021; 9:171.

49. Nóbrega DF, Fernández CE, Del Bel Cury AA, et al. Frequency of Fluoride Dentifrice Use and Caries Lesions Inhibition and Repair. Caries Res 2016;50(2): 133–40.

50. Francois P, Fouquet V, Attal JP, et al. Commercially Available Fluoride-Releasing Restorative Materials: A Review and a Proposal for Classification. Mater Basel Switz 2020;13(10):E2313.

51. Slimani A, Sauro S, Gatón Hernández P, et al. Commercially Available Ion-Releasing Dental Materials and Cavitated Carious Lesions: Clinical Treatment Options. Materials 2021;14(21):6272.

52. Braga RR. Calcium phosphates as ion-releasing fillers in restorative resin-based materials. Dent Mater 2019;35(1):3–14.

53. Bienek DR, Giuseppetti AA, Skrtic D. Amorphous calcium phosphate as bioactive filler in polymeric dental composites. London: IntechOpen; 2019.

54. Kasraei S, Haghi S, Valizadeh S, et al. Phosphate Ion Release and Alkalizing Potential of Three Bioactive Dental Materials in Comparison with Composite Resin. Int J Dent 2021;2021:5572569.

55. Monteiro JC, Stürmer M, Garcia IM, et al. Dental Sealant Empowered by 1,3,5-Tri Acryloyl Hexahydro-1,3,5-Triazine and α-Tricalcium Phosphate for Anti-Caries Application. Polymers 2020;12(4):E895.

56. Balhaddad AA, Kansara AA, Hidan D, et al. Toward dental caries: Exploring nanoparticle-based platforms and calcium phosphate compounds for dental restorative materials. Bioact Mater 2019;4(1):43–55.

57. Fei X, Li Y, Weir MD, et al. Novel pit and fissure sealant containing nano-CaF2 and dimethylaminohexadecyl methacrylate with double benefits of fluoride release and antibacterial function. Dent Mater Off Publ Acad Dent Mater 2020;36(9): 1241–53.

58. Mitwalli H, AlSahafi R, Alhussein A, et al. Novel rechargeable calcium fluoride dental nanocomposites. Dent Mater 2021. https://doi.org/10.1016/j.dental.2021. 12.022.

59. Baras BH, Melo MAS, Thumbigere-Math V, et al. Novel Bioactive and Therapeutic Root Canal Sealers with Antibacterial and Remineralization Properties. Mater Basel Switz 2020;13(5):E1096.

60. Sarikaya R, Song L, Yuca E, et al. Bioinspired multifunctional adhesive system for next generation bio-additively designed dental restorations. J Mech Behav Biomed Mater 2021;113:104135.

61. Albeshir EG, Balhaddad AA, Mitwalli H, et al. Minimally-invasive dentistry via dual-function novel bioactive low-shrinkage-stress flowable nanocomposites. Dent Mater Off Publ Acad Dent Mater 2021. https://doi.org/10.1016/j.dental. 2021.12.023. S0109-5641(21)00354-7.

62. Ibrahim MS, Balhaddad AA, Garcia IM, et al. pH-responsive calcium and phosphate-ion releasing antibacterial sealants on carious enamel lesions in vitro. J Dent 2020;97:103323.

63. Ibrahim MS, Balhaddad AA, Garcia IM, et al. Tooth sealing formulation with bacteria-killing surface and on-demand ion release/recharge inhibits early childhood caries key pathogens. J Biomed Mater Res B Appl Biomater 2020;108(8): 3217–27.

64. Hesaraki S, Karimi M, Nezafati N. The synergistic effects of SrF2 nanoparticles, YSZ nanoparticles, and poly-ε-l-lysin on physicomechanical, ion release, and antibacterial-cellular behavior of the flowable dental composites. Mater Sci Eng C 2020;109:110592.

65. Montoya C, Jain A, Londoño JJ, et al. Multifunctional Dental Composite with Piezoelectric Nanofillers for Combined Antibacterial and Mineralization Effects. ACS Appl Mater Inter 2021;13(37):43868–79.

66. Balhaddad AA, Garcia IM, Mokeem L, et al. Bifunctional Composites for Biofilms Modulation on Cervical Restorations. J Dent Res 2021;100(10):1063–71.

67. Abbassy MA, Bakry AS, Almoabady EH, et al. Characterization of a novel enamel sealer for bioactive remineralization of white spot lesions. J Dent 2021;109: 103663.

68. Ramadoss R, Padmanaban R, Subramanian B. Role of bioglass in enamel remineralization: Existing strategies and future prospects-A narrative review. J Biomed Mater Res B Appl Biomater 2022;110(1):45–66.

69. Jang JH, Lee MG, Ferracane JL, et al. Effect of bioactive glass-containing resin composite on dentin remineralization. J Dent 2018;75:58–64.

70. Lee MJ, Seo YB, Seo JY, et al. Development of a Bioactive Flowable Resin Composite Containing a Zinc-Doped Phosphate-Based Glass. Nanomater Basel Switz 2020;10(11):E2311.

71. Huang CT, Smith NR, Burgess JO, et al. In vitro inhibition of demineralization from bioglass-containing adhesive and composite. Am J Dent 2021;34(6):333–7.

72. Chiang YC, Wang YC, Kung JC, et al. Antibacterial silver-containing mesoporous bioglass as a dentin remineralization agent in a microorganism-challenged environment. J Dent 2021;106:103563.
73. Palza Cordero H, Castro Cid R, Diaz Dosque M, et al. Li-doped bioglass® 45S5 for potential treatment of prevalent oral diseases. J Dent 2021;105:103575.
74. Yao C, Ahmed MH, Li X, et al. Zinc-Calcium-Fluoride Bioglass-Based Innovative Multifunctional Dental Adhesive with Thick Adhesive Resin Film Thickness. ACS Appl Mater Inter 2020;12(27):30120–35.
75. Wang X, Huyang G, Palagummi SV, et al. High performance dental resin composites with hydrolytically stable monomers. Dent Mater Off Publ Acad Dent Mater 2018;34(2):228–37.
76. Bhadila G, Wang X, Zhou W, et al. Novel low-shrinkage-stress nanocomposite with remineralization and antibacterial abilities to protect marginal enamel under biofilm. J Dent 2020;99:103406.
77. Bhadila G, Menon D, Wang X, et al. Long-term antibacterial activity and cytocompatibility of novel low-shrinkage-stress, remineralizing composites. J Biomater Sci Polym Ed 2021;32(7):886–905.
78. Bhadila G, Wang X, Weir MD, et al. Low-shrinkage-stress nanocomposite: An insight into shrinkage stress, antibacterial, and ion release properties. J Biomed Mater Res B Appl Biomater 2021;109(8):1124–34.

Digital Technologies for Restorative Dentistry

Hidehiko Watanabe, DDS, MS*, Christopher Fellows, DDS, Hongseok An, DDS, MSD

KEYWORDS

- Direct and indirect digitization • Computer-aided design • Virtual design
- Computer-aided manufacturing • CAD/CAM materials • Implant digital impression
- Implant CAD/CAM

KEY POINTS

- Digitization of oral structure is the first step of computer-aided design/computer-aided manufacturing (CAD/CAM) dentistry. Practitioners need to know the pros and cons of direct and indirect digitization methods.
- Current technologies allow us to conduct virtual design of restorations supported by virtual simulation technologies, including smile design and a virtual articulator.
- Several different computer-aided manufacturing (CAM) methods can be selected by clinicians depending on the complexity and extent of clinical cases.
- The application of CAD/CAM to implant restorations is well established, and it is crucial to know the material types and properties of each abutment.

DIGITIZATION OF ORAL STRUCTURES

In order to use a digital workflow, oral structures must be converted into a 3-dimensional (3D) data format that can be processed by a computer. This digitization process is usually achieved by optically scanning them either directly or indirectly. The following section describes these 2 processes and highlights its advantages and disadvantages.

Direct Digitization

Teeth and other oral structures can be directly scanned using a hand-held intraoral scanner. This is often called digital impression or intraoral scanning. Intraoral scanning is widely used because it is time-saving and more patient friendly.[1]

The accuracy and convenience of this technology have been improved considerably during the last decade. Most of currently available studies concluded that the accuracy of intraoral scanning is comparable with that of conventional polyvinyl siloxane

Restorative Dentistry, Oregon Health & Science University, School of Dentistry, 2730 S Moody Avenue, Portland, OR 97201-5042, USA
* Corresponding author.
E-mail address: watanabh@ohsu.edu

Dent Clin N Am 66 (2022) 567–590
https://doi.org/10.1016/j.cden.2022.05.006
0011-8532/22/© 2022 Elsevier Inc. All rights reserved.

impressions and suitable for fabrication of single tooth restorations or short-span fixed dental prostheses (FDP).[2]

One of the limitations of intraoral scanning is that scanning larger areas requires merging of multiple images, and this may lead to a higher inaccuracy.[3] This progressive distortion tends to become more significant when scanning a longer distance. Therefore, full-arch intraoral scanning has a higher potential to create a larger discrepancy compared with conventional polyvinyl siloxane impressions.[2]

Another frequently mentioned limitation of intraoral scanning is its inability to capture movable tissue. Because accurate merging of multiple images can be achieved only if the shape of scanned objects does not change during scanning, intraoral scanning cannot be used predictably to make impressions for removable prostheses that require border molding (**Fig. 1**).

Indirect Digitization

When direct digitization is not indicated, indirect digitization can be achieved by scanning conventionally made impressions or stone casts using a laboratory scanner. This may be more time-consuming but it is a reliable way of achieving digitization as long as the impressions and casts are accurately made. Although accuracy of laboratory scanners is higher than that of intraoral scanners, dimensional distortions from impression materials and dental stones should be considered when evaluating accuracy of indirect digitization. Indirect digitization generates digital models with the accuracy that is comparable or superior to direct digitization depending on the properties and length of scanned oral structures.[4] Indirect digitization is still recommended over direct digitization for full-arch scanning when cross-arch accuracy is critical.[5] Indirect digitization may also be preferred when fabricating removable dental prostheses that include the movable part of oral mucosa or long-span splinted tooth or implant supported FDP.

Indirect digitization is commonly achieved by scanning stone casts. When using a laboratory scanner, objects are fixed on the table and the movements of light source and the table are precisely controlled by the scanner. As a result, the scanned images are directly registered to the internal coordinate system, and this does not rely on superimposition of images using overlapped areas. Early version of laboratory scanners project light to the objects only from a fixed angle. Some recent scanners have the capability of moving the objects during scanning, which allows the objects to be

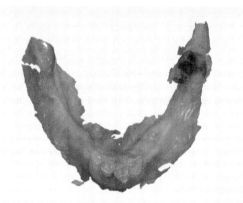

Fig. 1. Intraoral scanning of a long edentulous area may not be indicated when border molding is required.

scanned from different angles (**Fig. 2**). However, the range of motion is still restricted compared with that of hand-held intraoral scanners, and this makes it difficult to obtain a clear scan of certain areas such as undercuts and interproximal areas. If critical areas are missed, 2-step scanning technique can be used to obtain an accurate scan of the missed areas (**Fig. 3**A–C).

For some cases, a traditionally made impression can be scanned without fabricating a stone cast (**Fig. 4**A–C). It is possible only when the impression is relatively shallow without major undercuts around critical areas. Impressions of posterior area can often be more successfully scanned than those of anterior area. Accuracy of virtual models directly obtained by scanning a dental impression is known to be clinically acceptable.[6] Stone casts still need to be fabricated if physical try-in and adjustment of definitive restorations are desired.

Digital Scan Files

Once prepared teeth and other oral structures are successfully digitized, the digital image files are imported to computer-aided design (CAD) software to design dental prostheses. Most dental CAD/CAM systems have their own specific file format. If the same system is used for both scanning and designing, the system-specific file format may be used. If the CAD program does not accept the file format of the scanned image, the scanned image file should be converted to a general 3D file format, such as *.stl or *.ply, that the CAD software can accept. During this file conversion process, some data information, such as color or margin drawing, might be lost and the file size typically increases. Although using a closed or same system has advantages of being efficient and preserving full data, it still has limitations that it is not capable of expanding its workflow outside what the system allows and not able to communicate with other clinicians or technicians who are not equipped with the same system. For this reason, a closed system may be preferred when an efficient and repetitive execution of simple tasks is required (eg, chairside design and milling of 1-day restorations) and an open system may be preferred when more complex tasks are required (eg, commercial laboratory).

COMPUTER-AIDED DESIGN
Virtual Design

Once scanned images are imported to CAD software, virtual models are generated and prepared for design. Most CAD programs provide a design proposal based on

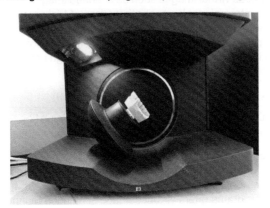

Fig. 2. Some recent laboratory scanners are capable of rotating the object and scanning it from different angles.

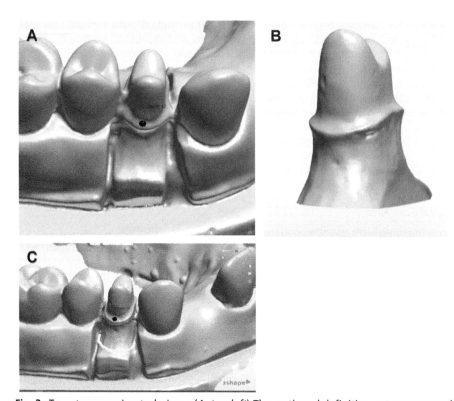

Fig. 3. Two-step scanning technique. (*A: top left*) The sectioned definitive cast was scanned using a laboratory scanner. The finish line was not clearly scanned. (*B: top right*) The prepared tooth was separately scanned. (*C: bottom left*) Two scanned images were merged to create the virtual working model.

the selected tooth form and surrounding structures such as adjacent and opposing teeth. The initial proposed design tends to be more satisfactory for single tooth restorations but virtual design of multiple restorations or extensive FDP may pose a significant challenge. Various virtual images such as scanned images of diagnostic models, interim prostheses, intraoral mock-up, or other types of trial prostheses can be useful when evaluating virtual design (**Fig. 5**A–C). Computer-aided design is a new tool that makes designing process more efficient. However, it does not change the conventional design criteria for dental prostheses. The basic design principles for dental prostheses should still be respected.

Virtual Simulation Technologies: Creating a Virtual Patient

Recent dental CAD programs are equipped with virtual simulation technology such as virtual smile design and virtual articulator to assist in creating ideal design.

Virtual smile design

Establishing harmonious positional relationship between teeth and other facial components has been emphasized as a critical part of prosthodontic treatment planning. Many dental CAD programs offers virtual esthetic simulation technology, often called virtual smile design or digital smile design, to help operators reorient migrated, malposed, or damaged teeth to the appropriate facial features.

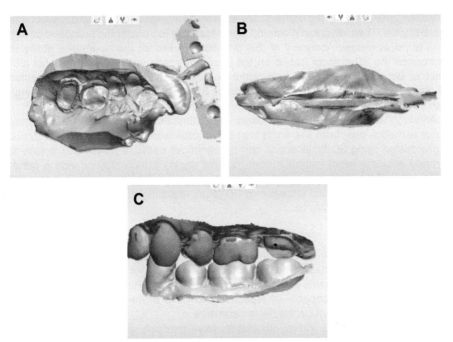

Fig. 4. Scanning a triple tray impression. (*A*: *top left*) Maxillary arch scan. Red spots indicate unscanned areas (*B*: *top right*) Maxillary and mandibular scans are merged. (*C*: *bottom left*) The merged image is reversed to generate the virtual working model.

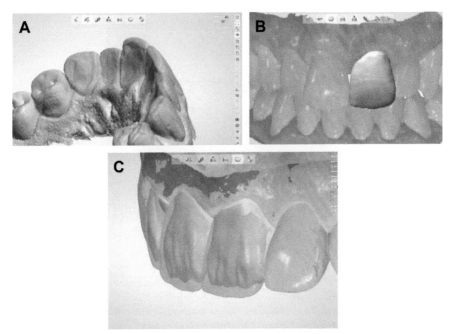

Fig. 5. Design references. (*A*: *top left*) Scan made before tooth preparation. (*B*: *top right*) Mirror image of the contralateral tooth. (*C*: *bottom left*) Diagnostic wax-up.

Virtual smile design in the earlier years used line drawings and a virtual caliper on the facial photos. Then, diagnostic wax-up was necessary to transfer the proposed design to a physical model. Accuracy of this procedure relies on the operator's ability to reproduce the 3D objects based on the drawings made on the 2-dimensional (2D) photos. Because recent virtual simulation technology allows direct superimposition of digital impressions to 2D facial photos or 3D facial scans, the proposed design can be transferred to the 3D model or final restorations with a higher precision.[7,8]

Although useful, 2D virtual smile design has a limitation that it allows evaluation of facial esthetics only from the angle that the photos were taken (**Fig. 6**A, B). Virtual smile design using 3D facial scans can be beneficial because it allows clinicians to virtually evaluate facial esthetics from multiple angles, which may provide a better perception of the esthetic impact of the planned treatment. It is expected that the use of this technology will increase as 3D facial scanning using smart phone apps are now available (**Fig. 7**A, B).

Virtual articulator

When a digital workflow is used, the virtual articulator replaces a traditional dental articulator. A virtual articulator is a computer software tool that is capable of reproducing the interarch relationship and simulating jaw movement. Recently, the dynamic virtual articulator that is capable of replicating function of mechanical articulators is available for most current dental design software.

Since first introduced, virtual articulators have gradually gained interest from researchers and clinicians in dentistry during the past decade; now it is considered as a necessary tool in digital dentistry, and many dental CAD/CAM programs currently include virtual articulator modules within their design system.

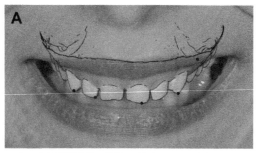

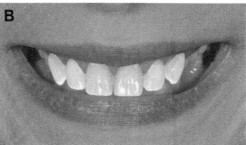

Fig. 6. A 2D virtual smile design. (*A: top*) Facial photo is aligned to a digital impression using common reference points. (*B: bottom*) Diagnostic design made on the digital impression can be evaluated on the facial photo.

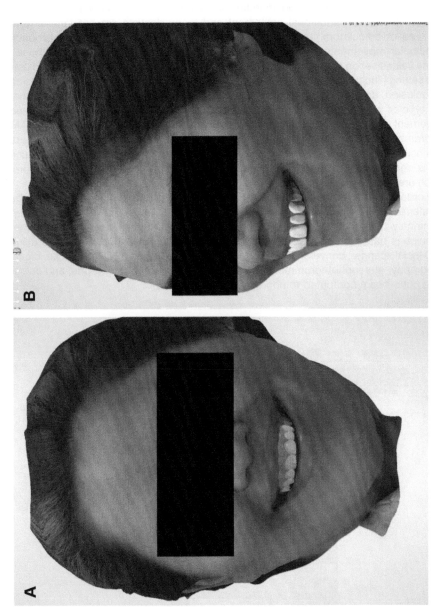

Fig. 7. A 3D virtual smile design. (*A: left*) Facial scan is aligned with the diagnostic digital impression. (*B: right*) Diagnostic design can be viewed from multiple angles to evaluate its esthetic impact.

There are currently 2 major types of virtual articulators—completely adjustable and mathematically simulated.[9] A completely adjustable articulator records and reproduces exact motion paths of the mandible using an electronic jaw registration system. This type of articulators may be indicated for complex cases where occlusion needs to be accurately assessed during mandibular movements but it is not widely used because it requires additional equipment and many dentists are not familiar with this type of articulators.[9] A mathematically simulated virtual articulator reproduce mandibular movements by mathematically calculating paths of movements based on the values set on the articulator. Depending on the articulator selected, the adjustable settings include Bennett angle, horizontal condylar inclination, vertical dimension of occlusion, and incisal table inclination (**Fig. 8**A–C). The main disadvantage is that this type of articulator is not capable of capturing and reproducing individualized movement of the patient. However, many commercially available dental CAD/CAM programs use this type of virtual articulator because it is more user friendly and less expensive.[9,10] Dentists are also more familiar with this type of articulators because this is considered as a digital equivalent of semiadjustable mechanical articulators, which are very commonly used.

In order to use the virtual articulator, the patient's maxilla and mandible need to be transferred to the virtual articulator. This step is often called virtual facebow transfer. Commonly used virtual facebow techniques include arbitrary mounting and other techniques based on cephalometric radiography, scanning extraoral markers using a 3D facial scanner, conversion of a series of photographs into a 3D facial scan, digital axiography, stereophotogrammetry, standardized extraoral photographs, and calculated cone-beam computed tomography (CBCT) (**Fig. 9**).[10]

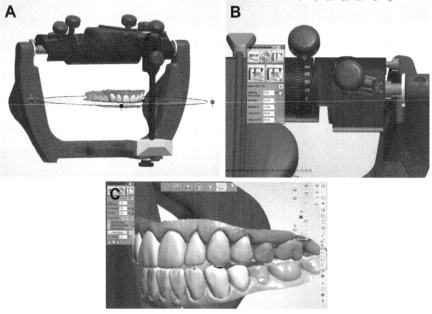

Fig. 8. Mathematically calculated semiadjustable articulator. (*A: top left*) mounted digital impressions. (*B: top right*) adjustable condylar settings. (*C: bottom left*) simulation of eccentric jaw movements.

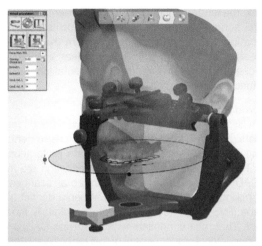

Fig. 9. Digital facebow transfer. Anatomic landmarks on a facial scan can be used to guide positioning the maxillary cast on the virtual articulator.

Most studies investigating accuracy of the virtual articulator focused on evaluating accuracy of static articulation. Although alignment method, arch length, type of the scanner, articulation methods, virtual articulation algorithm, and the use of mechanical articulators have been identified as influencing factors, most studies have reported that the accuracy of static articulation using the virtual articulator is clinically acceptable and comparable to a mechanical articulator.[11,12] Accuracy of dynamic virtual articulation, especially mathematically simulated articulation, has not been investigated as extensively as that of static virtual articulation. It was reported in the in-vitro study that eccentric movements on the mathematically simulated articulator showed the accuracy that is similar to that of the mechanical articulator and had less than 100 μm of deviations during dynamic movements.[13] Although this result seems promising, it is still recommended to use the virtual articulator as an additional diagnostic and treatment planning tool to the mechanical articulator, especially in complex cases involving alterations to the vertical dimension of occlusion, because the actual clinical application of dynamic virtual articulator involves many other variables and still requires further investigation.[10]

COMPUTER-AIDED MANUFACTURING
The Location of Production

Chairside production
The chairside production of restorations was introduced by the first Chair-side Economical Restoration of Esthetic Ceramic (CEREC) system in 1985.[14,15] In this method, a scanner, design software, and a milling unit were needed in the dental office, and nowadays it covers all fabrication steps, including sintering, crystallizing, or finishing, such as staining and glazing. This workflow is especially effective in a single restoration, and still, many practitioners may think of this system first when CAD/CAM dentistry is discussed. CEREC (Dentsply Sirona: Charlotte, North Carolina) and Planmeca (Planmeca: Helsinki, Finland) are the 2 most popular systems designed for chairside production in the market. Their current models are CEREC Primescan AC and Prinmemill, and Planmeca Emerald S and Planmeca PlanMill, respectively. In general, their designing software is simplified compared with the ones used in dental

laboratories. Because the fundamental steps for digital dentistry can be learned in this system, many dental schools introduced it because of its simplicity. Moreover, by managing the fabrication steps, practitioners can learn the importance of precision in each step, such as smooth tooth preparation, clear scanning, and appropriate designing steps. Those are important factors for the dental laboratory, and centralized fabrication is described as follows.

Dental laboratory production

This approach is similar to traditional communication with dental technicians. Dentists can send master casts produced from physical impressions to dental laboratories.[14,15] Then, laboratories digitally scan, design, and fabricate restorations using their own CAD/CAM devices. The advantages of laboratory fabrication are that dentists do not have to own the CAD/CAM devices, including intraoral scanners, computers with designing software, milling units, and firing ovens. When a dentist takes an impression with polyvinyl siloxane (PVS), many dental laboratories digitally fabricate a restoration from the master cast. That means dentists without having CAD/CAM technology are already using digital dentistry. Another benefit of this technique is that CAD/CAM restorations can be manually refined by trained laboratory technicians. Because chairside CAD/CAM units are not available in every dental office, digital laboratory restorations are the most popular format in current restorative dentistry. Another option in this category is that a dentist can also send the scanned digital impression to a laboratory. In this way, a dental office only needs to have an intraoral scanner in the CAD/CAM steps.

Centralized fabrication

This system connects satellite scanners in dental laboratories to a production center.[14,15] The production center produces restorations according to the data of designed restorations from laboratories, and then milled, or printed products are sent to the responsible laboratories. The advantage of this path is that dental laboratories can avoid installing costly milling units or 3D printers and focus on the final refinement of products. When complex cases such as full mouth reconstruction require multiple crowns and implants, or frameworks for partial dentures, outsourcing to a production center with the best equipment contributes to efficiency.

Subtractive or Additive Technique

Subtractive technique from a solid block

In this method, restorations are milled with diamond or carbide burs, depending on the material being milled. Typically, glass-ceramics are grinded with diamond burs.[16] However, zirconia or polymeric materials are milled with carbide burs. Dentsply Sirona recently modified the terminology in their subtractive approach in their software program, and "milling" is used for carbide burs, and "grinding" is used for the CAM with diamond burs. Using factory-fabricated ceramic or composite blocks in ideal conditions have consistent quality and are free from internal defects. Maximum strength of each material can be obtained in the subtractive fabrication.[17] However, a large portion of the material is wasted in this process, and a study reported that material loss could reach 90%.[18] Another drawback is that the size of milling burs limits the surface quality. Defective restorations due to the deterioration of milling burs can be a problem. **Fig. 10**A–D shows a clinical example of subtractive technique from a solid block.

Additive technique

There are 2 popular technologies for the additive technique in dentistry, including stereolithography (SLA) and direct metal laser sintering (DMLS).[19] The former is used for

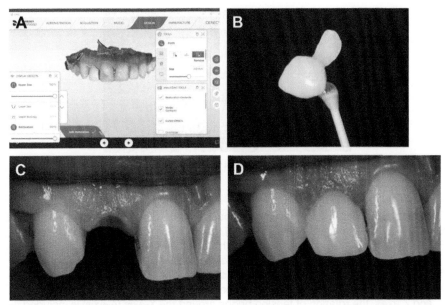

Fig. 10. Chairside production/subtractive manufacturing. (*A: top left*) Missing maxillary lateral incisor. (*B: top right*) A cantilever resin-bonded fixed dental prostheses was designed using CEREC software. (*C: bottom left*) A lithium disilicate restoration was milled and crystalized. (*D: bottom right*) Final restoration was bonded on the same day.

aligner fabrication, and the latter is applied for metal crowns and appliance frameworks (**Fig. 11**). The additive technique allows dental technicians and dentists to produce a solid 3D model from digital models created by a scanner and design software. In the additive manufacturing process, the models are built up by the sequential application of thin layers of material.[20] The additive technique can save material and express more complex geometries than subtractive methods.[20] However, currently additive fabrication is generally limited to polymeric and metallic.[14] There are several additive methods such as SLA, selective laser sintering, fused deposition modeling, DMLS, polyjet 3D printing, inkjet 3D printing, laminated object manufacturing, colorjet printing, electron beam melting, and multijet orienting that have a potential to solve challenges in complex surgical, prosthodontic, and orthodontic treatments.[19] A clinical case used a printed model is presented in **Fig. 12**A–F. Additive manufacturing is discussed further in "Additive Manufacturing" section.

Classification by the Number of Milling Axes

Three-axis devices
Examples: inLab (Dentsply Sirona: Charlotte, North Carolina), Lava (3M ESPE: St. Paul, Minneapolis), Cercon brain (DeguDent: Hanau Germany).

Three-axis devices can move milling burs to 3 axial directions denoted by X, Y, and Z values. This type of device can turn the component by 180° during the milling process of the external and intaglio surfaces of the restoration. These devices can be controlled relatively easily due to the simplified 3-axis and complete milling procedure with lower cost relative to the ones with a higher number of milling axes. However, 3-axis devices cannot mill subsections, axis divergences, and convergences.[16,17,21]

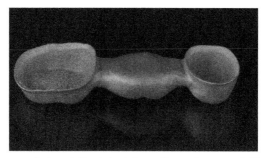

Fig. 11. Additively manufactured fixed dental prostheses framework (Co-Cr alloy).

Four-axis devices

Examples: Ceramill Mikro 4X (Amann Girrbach: Charlotte, North Carolina), Planmeca PlanMill 40 S (Planmeca: Helsinki, Finland), Zeno (Wieland-Imes: Hessen, Germany), Primemill (Dentsply Sirona: Charlotte, North Carolina)

Four-axis devices make a similar movement as the 3-axis milling process in that cutting burs or disks are used to produce the scanned or designed shape. However, the milling process is conducted with an additional axis in the 4-axis. In addition to the X, Y, and Z axes, the rotation of tension bridge around the X-axis (A-axis) is included as the fourth axis. A large vertical height displacement owing to the fourth axis enables to adjust bridges, and this device has the advantages of saving material and milling time.[16,17,21]

Five-axis devices

Examples: Versamill (Axsys Dental Solutions: Wixom, Michigan)

In 5-axis devices, the capability of rotation of milling spindle (5-axis) is added to the abovementioned axes of 4-axis machining. This fifth axis is located around the B-axis, rotating around the Y-axis. This results in the multidirectional rotation that helps produce complex geometry with subsections such as fixed partial dentures (FPDs) with converging abutment teeth or mesially tipped molar abutment.[16,17,21] It seems that the number of milling axes is not directly related to the quality of final restorations. The more milling axes, the higher the cost and the larger the device. In general, restorations with complex geometries require a milling unit with increased milling axes.[17] Dentists and technicians need to select milling units based on their practice types and the typical cases with which they deal because the digitalization process, data processing, and production process are more important than the milling devices in the quality of restorations.

Materials for Computer-Aided Manufacturing

Fasbinder and colleagues (2018) classified the chairside CAD/CAM blocks into 5 types **(Table 1)**. This classification may be different from the classification strictly based on ceramic material science but it is helpful for practitioners. They are resilient ceramics, composite, provisional, adhesive ceramics, high-strength ceramics, and zirconia.[22]

Adhesive ceramics

This material category was used first for CAD/CAM systems in the 1980s.[22] When the CAD/CAM technology was introduced, the only material available for restorations was traditional feldspathic ceramics. Examples of this material are CEREC Blocks (Dentsply Sirona, Charlotte, North Carolina), VITABLOCs Mark II (VITA Zahnfabrik: Yorba Linda, California), VITABLOCS RealLife Ceramic Blocks (VITA: Yorba Linda,

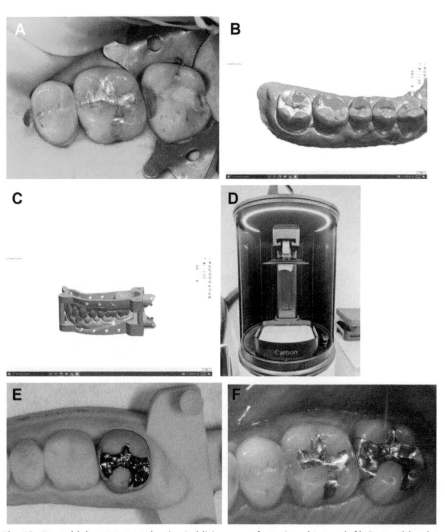

Fig. 12. Dental laboratory production/additive manufacturing. (*A: top left*) Cast gold onlay preparation. (*B: top right*) Designing a restoration. (*C: middle left*) Digital model. (*D: middle right*) Printing models with a carbon 3D printer. (*E: bottom left*) Cast gold fabrication on a printed model. (*F: bottom right*) Cast gold restoration delivery.

California), and VITABLOC TriLux Forte (VITA: Yorba Linda, California). This material is the most translucent and esthetic.[23] Although their flexural strength is relatively lower compared with other ceramics, one study reported 95% of the survival rate on premolar and molar crowns for 12 years.[24] Currently, this material is still used for veneers and partial veneer restorations. Leucite-reinforced ceramics was introduced in the late 1990s with increased strength and high translucency for anterior crowns, veneers, and posterior inlays/onlays. The survival rate of the CAD/CAM-generated leucite-reinforced ceramic restoration is high, and they are 94.6% and 97% for partial coverage posterior restorations.[25,26] However, after the introduction of lithium disilicate, the use of this material is decreasing. ProCAD (Karlsruhe, Germany) and Ivoclar Porcelain System (IPS) EmpressCAD (Ivoclar: Schaan, Liechtenstein) are included in this category.

Table 1
Classification of chairside CAD/CAM materials

Classification	Workflow	Material	Manufacturer
Resilient Ceramics	Grind/polish Mill/polish	Nanoceramic	Lava Ultimate (3M) CeraSmart (GC America: Alsip, Illinois) TetricCAD (Ivoclar: Schaan, Liechtenstein)
		PICN	Enamic (Vita: Bad Säckingen, Germany)
Composite		Bis-GMA	Paradigm MZ100 (3M: St. Paul, Minneapolis) Brilliant Crios (Coltene: Altstätten, Switzerland)
Provisional		PMMA	TelioCAD (Ivoclar: Schaan, Liechtenstein) Vita-CAD Temp (Vita: Bad Säckingen, Germany)
Adhesive ceramics	Grind/polish or stain and glaze	leucite-reinforced	IPS EmpressCAD (Ivoclar: Schaan, Liechtenstein)
		Feldspathic	Vita Mark II (Vita: Bad Säckingen, Germany) CEREC Blocks (Dentsply Sirona: Charlotte, North Carolina)
High-strength ceramics		Zinc-reinforced lithium silicate	Celtra Duo: Charlotte, North Carolina (Dentsply Sirona: Charlotte, North Carolina) Suprinity (Vita: Bad Säckingen, Germany)
	Grind/matrix fire	Advanced lithium disilicate	CEREC Tessera (Dentsply Sirona: Charlotte, North Carolina)
	Grind/crystallize	Lithium disilicate	IPS emaxCAD: Schaan, Liechtenstein (Ivoclar: Schaan, Liechtenstein)
Zirconia	Dry mill/sinter	Zirconia oxide	CEREC Zirconia+ (Dentsply Sirona: Charlotte, North Carolina) Katana Zirconia (Kuraray Noritake: Tokyo, Japan) 3M Chairdide Zirconia (3M: St. Paul, Minneapolis)

Abbreviation: GMA, bisphenol A-glycidyl methacrylate; IPS, Ivoclar Porcelain System; PICN, polymer infiltrated ceramic network; PMMA, Polymethyl methacrylate.

Resilient ceramics, composite, and provisional

These 3 categories cover polymeric CAD/CAM materials. Composite CAD/CAM blocks (Paradigm MZ100, 3M) were launched soon after introducing feldspathic blocks for inlays and onlays. Then, once the first Resilient Ceramics (LAVA Ultimate, 3M) was introduced in 2011, several similar materials were produced by manufacturers (Enamic Vita: Yorba Linda, California, Cerasamart GC: Tokyo, Japan, Shofu Block HC Shofu: Kyoto, Japan, TetricCAD Ivoclar: Schaan, Liechtenstein). This category of products is also called nanoceramics, hybrid ceramics, or polymer-infiltrated-ceramic network materials, and all contain a resin matrix in addition to inorganic refractory compounds such as porcelains, glasses, ceramics, and glass ceramics.[22,23]

The advantages of this product are that its milled margins are smoother than glass ceramics, and it does not require a firing process. Although overall physical properties are inferior to ceramic materials, positive laboratory evaluations have been reported. Debonding was considered to be a problem initially. However, after proper bonding protocol, including pretreatment with aluminum oxide air-particle abrasion was provided to clinicians, several studies have reported acceptable to excellent survival rates (85.7% for 2 years, 97% for 3 years, 95.6% for 3 years).[27–29] Some manufacturers offer the option of polymethyl methacrylate (PMMA) provisional blocks. They are used for long-term provisional restorations (Telio CAD, Ivoclar Vivadent, VITA CAD-Temp MultiColor Blocks, VITA: Yorba Linda, California). Those products have advantages in esthetics and physical strength compared with conventional PMMA provisional restorations.

High-strength ceramics
Lithium disilicate (IPS emaxCAD: Schaan, Liechtenstein, Ivoclar Vivadent), zinc-reinforced lithium silicate (Celtra Duo: Charlotte, North Carolina, Dentsply Sirona, Suprinity, Vita: Yorba Linda, California), and advanced lithium disilicate (CEREC Tessera, Dentsply Sirona) are in this group. High-strength ceramics are the most popular materials for chair-side CAD/CAM restorations. The flexural strength of lithium disilicate is about 400 to 500 MPa, and clinical studies showed a survival rate of 97% for 2 years and 99% clinical survival rate at 5 years.[30,31] The advantages of this product are its physical strength enough for most posterior crowns, translucency as glass ceramics, and relatively easy finishing process, including polishing, staining, and glazing. However, it requires a 2-step firing, and the newly introduced advanced lithium disilicate (CEREC Tessera) also requires a 2-step firing process. The manufacturer's laboratory data showed 700 MPa of biaxial flexural strength for CEREC Tessera. Although long-term clinical data are not available, this material could be applied for stress-bearing molars.

Zirconia
CEREC Zirconia+ (Dentsply Sirona: Charlotte, North Carolina), Katana Zirconia (Kuraray Noritake: Tokyo, Japan), and 3M Chairdide Zirconia (3M) are in this category. Full contoured zirconia is the newest material for chair-side CAD/CAM restorations. The flexural strength of more translucent 5 mol% and 4 mol% zirconia materials are approximately 700 MPa and 900 MPa, respectively.[22] Due to the high strength, the minimal occlusal reduction can be 0.6 to 1 mm, depending on the zirconia products. However, there is no current evidence for long-term clinical performance of chair-side zirconia restorations.

CAD/CAM TECHNOLOGY IN IMPLANT DENTISTRY
Implant Digital Impression with Intraoral Scanners

Although the evidence on the accuracy of intraoral digital impressions for dental implants is limited, there is enough information to conclude that digital impressions are at least as accurate as analog impressions for fabrication of single unit implant restorations and short span implant FDP.[32,33] The accuracy of the dental implant scan is dependent on the intraoral scanner (IOS) used,[32,34] the design and material of the intraoral scan body (ISB),[35–37] the number and relative position of the dental implant fixture(s),[32,35] as well as the scanning protocol.[36,37] Some studies have shown that lighting conditions, operator experience, and implant angulation may also affect the accuracy of an implant scan.[32] The ISB (**Fig. 13**) is a critical component for obtaining an accurate implant scan, and it has been shown that different ISB designs perform

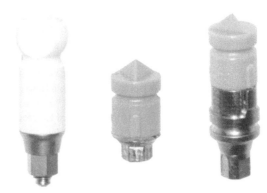

Fig. 13. Intraoral scan bodies.

best under specific conditions. Therefore, clinicians should expect to have multiple ISBs that work with their IOS systems for best results in all clinical situations.

Implant CAD/CAM Restoration Design

Recent advances in CAD/CAM manufacturing techniques and dental materials have expanded options for dental implant restoration fabrication that rival traditional fabrication methods in terms of restoration survival, esthetics, and biocompatibility.[32] Moreover, digital implant impression combined with CAD/CAM manufacturing has shown to be more time efficient and less costly than traditional fabrication methods and one that has been shown to be preferred by patients.[38]

CAM/CAM techniques may be used to fabricate custom implant abutments and crowns from various materials such as titanium, zirconia, and polyetheretherketone (PEEK). Although many of these CAD/CAM dental implant restoration designs have been shown to compare favorably to traditionally fabricated porcelain-fused-to-metal (PFM) and full gold restorations fabricated with gold University of California at Los Angeles (UCLA) abutments using analog techniques, research on these implant restoration designs is limited and there are ongoing concerns with the breakdown of the bonded interface(s) within the restoration.[39,40]

Titanium base hybrid restoration

Stock titanium base abutments are often used as the substructure for single unit, multiple unit, and full arch implant restorations (**Fig. 14**A). The titanium base serves as an interface or connection between the implant fixture and an implant restoration. The titanium base abutment is typically bonded to the restoration outside of the mouth, creating a custom screw retained "hybrid" restoration (see **Fig. 14**B). Blocks with predrilled holes are commonly used for the fabrication of single unit "hybrid" restorations using these stock titanium base abutments (see **Fig. 14**C). Multiple unit FDPs and full arch hybrid prosthesis may also incorporate titanium base abutments into the restoration design. Common materials used in the fabrication of these "hybrid" implant restorations are zirconia, lithium disilicate, PEEK, and PMMA. The screw channel does not seem to affect the longevity of hybrid restorations made from monolithic zirconia or lithium disilicate.[40–42] Screw access channels have been shown to affect the longevity of restorations made of PEEK and some composite materials, and as such are not recommended for long-term use.[40] Although zirconia and lithium disilicate ""hybrid" dental implant restorations using titanium base abutments have been shown to compare favorably to traditionally fabricated PFM and full gold restorations fabricated with gold UCLA abutments using analog techniques, there are ongoing

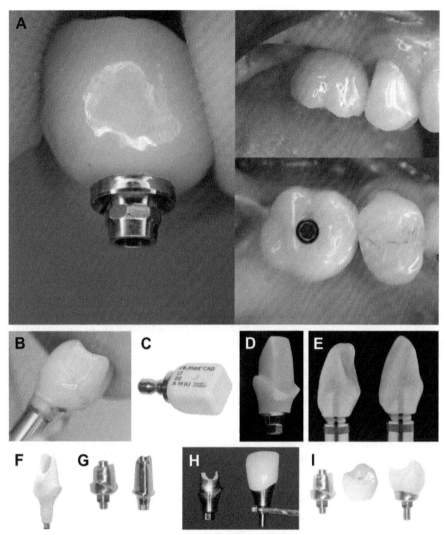

Fig. 14. Titanium base hybrid restoration. (*A*) Stock titanium base abutment. (*B*) Custom screw retained "hybrid" restoration. (*C*) CAD/CAM block. (*D*) Ustomized metal/ceramic hybrid abutment. (*E*) Restoration cemented to the custom hybrid abutment. (*F*) One-piece all zirconia abutment. (*G*) Titanium custom abutment. (*H*) Zirconia and zirconia/titanium base hybrid abutment. (*I*) Hybrid implant restoration using a custom base abutment.

concerns about the breakdown of the bonded interface between the titanium base abutment and the crown.[39,43] One of the main advantages of the titanium base hybrid restoration design is the ability to scan the dental implant and provide a screw-retained implant supported restoration in the same appointment.

Implant CAD/CAM Abutment Design

CAD/CAM is also used in the fabrication of custom implant abutments. These custom abutments may serve as the substructure for a screw-retained hybrid crown, or serve as the abutment for a cement-retained abutment supported restoration. The term custom base is commonly used when the final restoration design is a hybrid screw-retained crown.

Titanium base hybrid abutment

A stock titanium base abutment can also be used for fabrication of a customized metal/ceramic hybrid abutment (see **Fig. 14**D). With this design, a "meso" abutment is milled and bonded to the titanium base. A screw-retained crown can then be fabricated and bonded to the custom hybrid abutment, resulting in a hybrid screw retained restoration, or a restoration can be cemented to the custom hybrid abutment intraorally if a cement-retained crown is indicated (see **Fig. 14**E). Common materials for custom hybrid abutments are zirconia and lithium disilicate, which rival the mechanical stability of full contour custom titanium abutments, and offer improved esthetics.[42,44] Although reenforced PEEK shows promising in Vitro results for use as a hybrid abutment material, further investigation is needed.[45] Longevity of the bonding interfaces with hybrid abutment restorations are of concern,[39,44] and further studies are needed to evaluate debonding in clinical situations. From the studies that are available, lithium disilicate seems to have fewer debonding problems than zirconia.[39]

Zirconia CAD/CAM abutments

One-piece all zirconia abutments have been explored as an option for use in implant restoration, mainly for esthetic reasons (see **Fig. 14**F). Although studies are limited, full zirconia abutments have been shown to be more prone to fracture, especially in narrow diameter implant designs.[39,44] Zirconia abutments have also been shown to wear the implant fixture connection, leaching titanium and zirconia particles into the peri-implant tissues.[39,44] Titanium and titanium base hybrid abutments seem to have superior resistance to fracture, with esthetics that rival those made from full Zirconia.[39,41] Therefore, full Zirconia abutments should be used with caution, and limited in their use.

Titanium CAD/CAM abutments

Titanium custom abutments are one of the most commonly used substructures for dental implant restoration (see **Fig. 14**G). One of the drawbacks of titanium abutments is the propensity for gray shadowing of the peri-implant tissues, especially with thin tissue phenotypes. Titanium nitride (gold hue) abutments offer an excellent esthetic alternative to Zirconia and Zirconia/titanium base hybrid abutments (see **Fig. 14**H). These gold hue titanium abutments have much better fracture resistance than Zirconia, have similar esthetic scores, and there is no worry about the Zirconia meso abutment debonding from the titanium base as with the zirconia hybrid abutments.[39] A hybrid restoration made from a custom CAD/CAM titanium base abutment with a bonded lithium disilicate crown seems to be the most stable of the CAD/CAM implant restoration designs.[39]

Hybrid crowns using custom base abutments

Hybrid implant restorations using a custom base abutment is similar in design to the stock titanium base hybrid implant restoration, with some notable differences (see **Fig. 14**I). As with the stock titanium base hybrid restorations, common materials for fabrication of the crown for use with custom abutments/bases are zirconia and lithium disilicate. Although studies have shown little clinical differences between these 2 materials in their monolithic form with regards to fracture resistance and chipping, a greater risk of debonding has been shown with zirconia.[39] Predrilled blocks for screw retention of hybrid implant restorations using custom base abutments are not commercially available because they are for stock titanium base hybrid restorations.

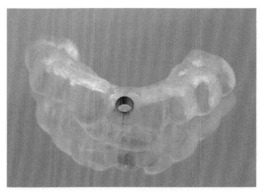

Fig. 15. Printed implant surgical guide with metal surgical sleeve.

Therefore, screw access channel has to be manually placed in the restoration after milling and bonded in place in the laboratory or chairside for a "hybrid" screw-retained restoration. The screw channel in the restoration may be eliminated, and the crown can be cemented directly in the patient's mouth for a cement-retained restoration. There seems to be no difference in the survivability of the "hybrid" screw-retained restoration when compared with the cement-retained restoration using this CAD/CAM protocol.[42] The screw-retained "hybrid" restorations have the advantage of retrievability and reduced soft tissue complications when compared with intraorally cemented or bonded abutment supported restorations.

Advances in CAD/CAM technology and improvements in restorative materials have resulted in many new implant restoration designs available to clinicians. Although long-term studies evaluating the success and survival of these implant restoration designs are lacking, enough information is available to conclude that many of these designs offer a reasonable alternative to traditionally fabricated implant restorations using cast-to-gold abutments. A hybrid restoration made from a custom CAD/CAM titanium abutment with a bonded lithium disilicate crown seems to give good esthetic results, good fracture resistance, and a reduced chance of debonding.

Additive Manufacturing

Additive manufacturing of dental appliances and restorations is rapidly becoming more commonplace as advances in additive dental materials and hardware technology improve. Additive manufacture is commonly used for some applications, such as printing of dental models, whereas additive manufacturing of dental restorations is still not as common as subtractive methods.

Additive manufacturing of polymer-based dental appliances
Additive manufacturing of dental polymers has been shown to be an efficient, accurate, and cost-effective process for fabrication of dental appliances such as occlusal guards, implant surgical guides, dental models, custom impression trays, and even complete dentures. One of the most common methods of polymer printing is via a process called SLA. SLA involves a laser that cures light-activated polymers in cross-sectional layers in a layer-by-layer approach to build up a 3D object. Other methods of additive manufacture using dental polymers include material jetting, material extrusion, and digital light processing.

Occlusal Guards/Splints, Surgical Guides, Printed Models, and Complete Dentures
Although a very limited number of studies on printed occlusal splints are available in the literature, initial findings on 3D printed occlusal splint wear and fracture resistance is promising.[46,47]

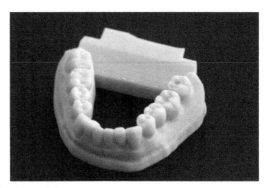

Fig. 16. Printed dental model.

The 3D printing of dental implant surgical guides (**Fig. 15**) has quickly become a routine part of a digital implant dentistry workflow. Implant planning software allows for virtual implant planning and placement and generates a file for surgical guide printing. Guides are commonly printed from a light cure resin with the addition of metal "surgical sleeves" into the printed guide. The accuracy of implant placement using these printed guides has been shown to be better than implant placement using conventional protocols.[48] Similarly, published studies have reported that the digital models are as reliable as traditional plaster casts, with high accuracy, reliability, and reproducibility[49] (**Fig. 16**).

CAD/CAM denture fabrication often times involves a combination of both analog and digital techniques. A conventional denture impression is obtained and digitized. Denture bases are printed and jaw relation records obtained. CAD is used for a virtual denture set up, and a try-in denture can then printed or milled. One of the advantages of printing try-in dentures is that multiple variations of the dentures may be printed to help determine which of the variations will be most acceptable to the patient. Once the try-in denture is verified in the patient's mouth, a final denture can then be printed or milled from the same file. As additive materials for printing dentures improve, this approach will undoubtedly become more common in the denture fabrication process.

Additive manufacturing of dental polymers for dental applications has a promising future. The development of protocols using a complete digital workflow for prosthetic dental disciplines are ongoing. Additive manufacturing will undoubtedly continue to play a significant role in these protocols in the future.

Additive manufacturing of metal restorations and ceramic restorations

Metal restorations can be additively manufactured using powder bed fusion technology. Commonly used powder bed fusion technologies include selective laser sintering, selective laser melting, and electron beam melting.[50] With the recent advancement in metal printing technology, a variety of metal alloys, such as titanium, high-noble, noble, and nonprecious metal alloys, are used for additive manufacturing of metal restorations. The physical properties of additively manufactured metal restorations have been investigated and shown promising results. Studies have shown that accuracy and strength of additively manufactured metal restorations are comparable to those of milled or cast metal restorations.[51,52] However, additively manufactured metal objects tend to be porous and rough. For this reason, additively manufacturing is typically used to fabricate metal frameworks or copings that are covered with ceramic or other materials.[53] Although subtractive manufacturing is more commonly used to fabricate metal restorations, it is expected that the use of additive manufacturing technology for metal restorations will increase. The advantages of additive manufacturing include the ability to reproduce complex geometry and reduced time and cost when compared with subtractive manufacturing.[54]

It is also possible to fabricate dental ceramic restorations using additive manufacturing but it is still in nascent stage. Additively manufactured zirconia restorations are mostly studied among different types of ceramic restorations. Additively manufactured zirconia restorations are not currently used for patient care as their physical properties and qualities are not as great as those of milled zirconia restorations. However, they have been studied as a potential alternative in experimental settings and have shown some promising outcomes.[55,56] With more advancement in additive technology and material science, additive manufacturing might become more popular in a near future.

SUMMARY AND FUTURE DIRECTIONS

Although intraoral scanners and CAD/CAM systems for restorative procedures have become approachable to beginners, faster, and more sophisticated in the last decade, the improvement of digital dentistry has the potential to change several aspects, including orthodontics, surgery, removable prosthesis, patient communications and management, dental education, and clinical research. It is also possible to send scanners to patients who live in underserved communities and have them scan self-scan for aligner fabrication or diagnostic purposes.[57] The digital data can be used for computer-assisted surgery and tissue-engineered scaffolds. Additive manufacturing is expected to play a significant role in developing new materials. It may be able to produce the complex color gradients of ceramic restorations mimicking natural tooth appearance, which is challenging for monolithic milled restorations.[57] Further improvement in digital dentistry is beneficial for clinicians, patients, researchers, and educators.

CLINICS CARE POINTS

- Direct and indirect digitization technique should be carefully selected considering type of restoration and clinical scenario.
- Virtual simulation technologies can be used to improve computer-aided design of dental restorations.
- Various digital workflows and materials are available for computer-aided manufacturing of dental restorations. Clinicians may choose the optimal workflow based on available resources and clinical scenarios.
- In combination with newer materials, CAD/CAM-generated implant restorations have become popular. Although previous studies showed promising outcomes, more studies are necessary to fully understand their clinical performance.

DISCLOSURE

The authors do not have any conflicts of interest to disclose.

REFERENCES

1. Schepke U, Meijer HJ, Kerdijk W, et al. Digital versus analog complete-arch impressions for single-unit premolar implant crowns: Operating time and patient preference. J Prosthet Dent 2015;114(3):403–6.e1.

2. Ahlholm P, Sipilä K, Vallittu P, et al. Digital versus conventional impressions in fixed prosthodontics: a review. J Prosthodont 2018;27(1):35–41.

3. Güth JF, Runkel C, Beuer F, et al. Accuracy of five intraoral scanners compared to indirect digitalization. Clin Oral Investig 2017;21(5):1445–55.

4. Quaas S, Loos R, Rudolph H, et al. Randomized controlled trial comparing direct intraoral digitization and extraoral digitization after impression taking. Int J Prosthodont 2015;28(1):30–2.

5. Wesemann C, Muallah J, Mah J, et al. Accuracy and efficiency of full-arch digitalization and 3D printing: a comparison between desktop model scanners, an intraoral scanner, a CBCT model scan, and stereolithographic 3D printing. Quintessence Int 2017;48(1):41–50.

6. Gül Amuk N, Karsli E, Kurt G. Comparison of dental measurements between conventional plaster models, digital models obtained by impression scanning and plaster model scanning. Int Orthod 2019;17(1):151–8.

7. Coachman C, Georg R, Bohner L, et al. Chairside 3D digital design and trial restoration workflow. J Prosthet Dent 2020;124(5):514–20.

8. Lin WS, Harris BT, Phasuk K, et al. Integrating a facial scan, virtual smile design, and 3D virtual patient for treatment with CAD-CAM ceramic veneers: a clinical report. J Prosthet Dent 2018;119(2):200–5.

9. Koralakunte PR, Aljanakh M. The role of virtual articulator in prosthetic and restorative dentistry. J Clin Diagn Res 2014;8(7):ZE25–8.

10. Lepidi L, Galli M, Mastrangelo F, et al. Virtual articulators and virtual mounting procedures: where do we stand? J Prosthodont 2021;30(1):24–35.

11. Edher F, Hannam AG, Tobias DL, et al. The accuracy of virtual interocclusal registration during intraoral scanning. J Prosthet Dent 2018;120(6):904–12.

12. Wong KY, Esguerra RJ, Chia VAP, et al. Three-dimensional accuracy of digital static interocclusal registration by three intraoral scanner systems. J Prosthodont 2018;27(2):120–8.

13. Hsu MR, Driscoll CF, Romberg E, et al. Accuracy of dynamic virtual articulation: trueness and precision. J Prosthodont 2019;28(4):436–43.

14. Abdullah A, Muhammed F, Zheng B, et al. An overview of computer aided design/computer aided manufacturing (CAD/CAM) in restorative dentistry. J Dental Mater Tech 2018;7(1):1–10.

15. Essa HAA. CAD/CAM in prosthodontics: a gate to the future. Int J Appl Dent Sci 2019;5(3):394–7.

16. Patil M, Kambale S, Patil A, et al. Digitalization in Dentistry: CAD/CAM -A Review. Acta Scientific Dental Sciences 2018;2(1):12–6.

17. Sriram S, Shankari V, Chacko Y. Computer aided designing/computer aided manufacturing in dentistry (CAD/CAM) – A review. Int J Curr Res Rev 2018; 10(20):20–4.

18. Strub JR, Rekow ED, Witkowski S. Computer-aided design and fabrication of dental restorations: current systems and future possibilities. J Am Dent Assoc 2006;137(9):1289–96.

19. Javaid M, Haleem A. Current status and applications of additive manufacturing in dentistry: a literature-based review. J Oral Biol Craniofac Res 2019;9(3):179–85.

20. Kessler A, Hickel R, Reymus M. 3D printing in dentistry-state of the art. Oper Dent 2020;45(1):30–40.

21. Abdulla M, Ali H, Jamel R. CAD-CAM technology: a literature review. Al-Rafidain Dental J 2020;20(1):95–113.

22. Fasbinder DJ. A review of chairside CAD/CAM materials. J Cosmet Dentistry 2018;34(3):65–74.

23. Blatz MB, Conejo J. The current state of chairside digital dentistry and materials. Dent Clin North Am 2019;63(2):175–97.
24. Otto T, Mörmann WH. Clinical performance of chairside CAD/CAM feldspathic ceramic posterior shoulder crowns and endocrowns up to 12 years. Int J Comput Dent 2015;18(2):147–61.
25. Nejatidanesh F, Amjadi M, Akouchekian M, et al. Clinical performance of CEREC AC Bluecam conservative ceramic restorations after five years–A retrospective study. J Dent 2015;43(9):1076–82.
26. Guess PC, Strub JR, Steinhart N, et al. All-ceramic partial coverage restorations–midterm results of a 5-year prospective clinical splitmouth study. J Dent 2009; 37(8):627–37.
27. Zimmermann M, Koller C, Reymus M, et al. Clinical evaluation of indirect particle-filled composite resin CAD/CAM partial crowns after 24 months. J Prosthodont 2018;27(8):694–9.
28. Lu T, Peng L, Xiong F, et al. A 3-year clinical evaluation of endodontically treated posterior teeth restored with two different materials using the CEREC AC chairside system. J Prosthet Dent 2018;119(3):363–8.
29. Spitznagel FA, Scholz KJ, Vach K, et al. Monolithic polymer-infiltrated ceramic network CAD/CAM single crowns: three-year mid-term results of a prospective clinical study. Int J Prosthodont 2020;33(2):160–8.
30. Reich S, Fischer S, Sobotta BAJ, et al. A preliminary study on the short-term efficacy of chairside computer-aided design/computer-assisted manufacturing-generated posterior lithium disilicate crowns. Int J Prosthodont 2010;23 3:214–6.
31. Fasbinder DJDJ, Heys D, Neiva GF. Five-year clinical evaluation of lithium disilicate chair-side CAD/CAM crowns. J Dent Res 2015;94:64–74. Special Issue A.
32. Michelinakis G, Apostolakis D, Kamposiora P, et al. The direct digital workflow in fixed implant prosthodontics: a narrative review. BMC Oral Health 2021;21(1):37.
33. Marques S, Ribeiro P, Falcão C, et al. Digital impressions in implant dentistry: a literature review. Int J Environ Res Public Health 2021;18(3):1020.
34. Imburgia M, Logozzo S, Hauschild U, et al. Accuracy of four intraoral scanners in oral implantology: a comparative in vitro study. BMC Oral Health 2017;17(1):92.
35. Fluegge T, Att W, Metzger M, et al. A novel method to evaluate precision of optical implant impressions with commercial scan bodies-an experimental approach. J Prosthodont 2017;26(1):34–41.
36. Mizumoto RM, Yilmaz B, McGlumphy EA Jr, et al. Accuracy of different digital scanning techniques and scan bodies for complete-arch implant-supported prostheses. J Prosthet Dent 2020;123(1):96–104.
37. Motel C, Kirchner E, Adler W, et al. Impact of different scan bodies and scan strategies on the accuracy of digital implant impressions assessed with an intraoral scanner: an in vitro study. J Prosthodont 2020;29(4):309–14.
38. Joda T, Brägger U. Digital vs. conventional implant prosthetic workflows: a cost/time analysis. Clin Oral Implants Res 2015;26(12):1430–5.
39. Pitta J, Hjerppe J, Burkhardt F, et al. Mechanical stability and technical outcomes of monolithic CAD/CAM fabricated abutment-crowns supported by titanium bases: an in vitro study. Clin Oral Implants Res 2021;32(2):222–32.
40. Preis V, Hahnel S, Behr M, et al. In-vitro fatigue and fracture testing of CAD/CAM-materials in implant-supported molar crowns. Dent Mater 2017;33(4):427–33.
41. Zacher J, Bauer R, Strasser T, et al. Laboratory performance and fracture resistance of CAD/CAM implant-supported tooth-coloured anterior FDPs. J Dent 2020; 96:103326.

42. Pitta J, Hicklin SP, Fehmer V, et al. Mechanical stability of zirconia meso-abutments bonded to titanium bases restored with different monolithic all-ceramic crowns. Int J Oral Maxillofac Implants 2019;34(5):1091–7.

43. DuVall NB, DeReis SP, Vandewalle KS. Fracture strength of various titanium-based, CAD-CAM and PFM implant crowns. J Esthet Restor Dent 2021;33(3):522–30.

44. Sadowsky SJ. Has zirconia made a material difference in implant prosthodontics? A review. Dent Mater 2020;36(1):1–8.

45. Atsü SS, Aksan ME, Bulut AC. Fracture resistance of titanium, zirconia, and ceramic-reinforced polyetheretherketone implant abutments supporting CAD/CAM monolithic lithium disilicate ceramic crowns after aging. Int J Oral Maxillofac Implants 2019;34(3):622–30.

46. Lutz AM, Hampe R, Roos M, et al. Fracture resistance and 2-body wear of 3-dimensional-printed occlusal devices. J Prosthet Dent 2019;121(1):166–72. Epub 2018 Jun 29. PMID: 30647000.

47. Berli C, Thieringer FM, Sharma N, et al. Comparing the mechanical properties of pressed, milled, and 3D-printed resins for occlusal devices. J Prosthet Dent 2020;124(6):780–6. Epub 2020 Jan 17. PMID: 31955837.

48. Yeung M, Abdulmajeed A, Carrico CK, et al. Accuracy and precision of 3D-printed implant surgical guides with different implant systems: an in vitro study. J Prosthet Dent 2020;123(6):821–8. https://doi.org/10.1016/j.prosdent.2019.05.027. Epub 2019 Oct 23. PMID: 31653399.

49. Revilla-León M, Özcan M. Additive manufacturing technologies used for processing polymers: current status and potential application in prosthetic dentistry. J Prosthodont 2019;28:146–58.

50. Revilla-León M, Meyer MJ, Özcan M. Metal additive manufacturing technologies: literature review of current status and prosthodontic applications. Int J Comput Dent 2019;22(1):55–67.

51. Tamac E, Toksavul S, Toman M. Clinical marginal and internal adaptation of CAD/CAM milling, laser sintering, and cast metal ceramic crowns. J Prosthet Dent 2014;112(4):909–13.

52. Takaichi A, Suyalatu, Nakamoto T, et al. Microstructures and mechanical properties of Co-29Cr-6Mo alloy fabricated by selective laser melting process for dental applications. J Mech Behav Biomed Mater 2013;21:67–76.

53. Alammar A, Kois JC, Revilla-León M, et al. Additive manufacturing technologies: current status and future perspectives. J Prosthodont 2022;31(S1):4–12.

54. Koutsoukis T, Zinelis S, Eliades G, et al. Selective laser melting technique of Co-Cr dental alloys: a review of structure and properties and comparative analysis with other available techniques. J Prosthodont 2015;24(4):303–12.

55. Methani MM, Revilla-León M, Zandinejad A. The potential of additive manufacturing technologies and their processing parameters for the fabrication of all-ceramic crowns: a review. J Esthet Restor Dent 2020;32(2):182–92.

56. Revilla-León M, Meyer MJ, Zandinejad A, et al. Additive manufacturing technologies for processing zirconia in dental applications. Int J Comput Dent 2020;23(1):27–37.

57. Rekow ED. Digital dentistry: the new state of the art—Is it disruptive or destructive? Dental Mater 2020;36(1):9–24.

Advances in Ceramics for Dental Applications

Atais Bacchi, DDS, MS, PhD[a],*, Paulo Francisco Cesar, DDS, MS, PhD[b]

KEYWORDS

- Y-TZP • Zirconia • Lithium-disilicate • Glass-ceramic • CAD-CAM • 3-D printing
- Strength • Wear

KEY POINTS

- Ceramic materials have been improved in terms of structural strength and optical properties, which in association with their excellent chemical stability culminates in optimal restorative materials.
- The development of color gradients and strength-graded ceramic blocks, as well as their diverse translucencies, provided an important advance for the production of computer-aided design–computer-aided manufacturing (CAD–CAM) restorations.
- The development of three-dimensional-printed ceramic restorations is emerging and seems to be promising.

INTRODUCTION

Ceramic materials have been widely and increasingly used for dental restorations because of their excellent esthetic appearance (adequately mimicking dental structures), good chemical stability (which plays a major role in the challenging oral environment in terms of pH, temperature, staining, etc.), and relatively high mechanical strength to resist occlusal forces without fracturing or wearing.[1] Since dental ceramics started to be more efficiently used in the early 1960s as veneering materials for metallic frameworks, several improvements have been made to their composition and processing methods, causing a significant impact on properties and clinical indications.

The aim of this review is to depict the most promising dental ceramics currently available in the dental market, focusing on their composition, commercial presentation, key properties, clinical indication, and processing methods.

---

[a] Post-Graduate Program in Dentistry, Paulo Picanço School of Dentistry, Rua Joaquim Sá 900, Fortaleza, Ceará 60325-218, Brazil; [b] Department of Biomaterials and Oral Biology, University of São Paulo – USP. Av Prof Lineu Prestes, 2227. Cidade Universitária, São Paulo, São Paulo 05508-000, Brazil
* Corresponding author.
E-mail address: atais_bacchi@yahoo.com.br

Dent Clin N Am 66 (2022) 591–602
https://doi.org/10.1016/j.cden.2022.05.007
0011-8532/22/© 2022 Elsevier Inc. All rights reserved.

The Materials

The current ceramic materials are classified in this review in three main groups according to their composition: glass-ceramics, polycrystalline ceramics, and polymer-infiltrated ceramic networks (PICNs).

GLASS-CERAMICS

Glass-ceramics are composed of a relevant amount of vitreous phase reinforced by crystals. The crystalline phase type and content in their microstructure directly affect the glass-ceramic's properties, such as strength and translucency.[2] The glassy phase present in these materials is responsible for the strong bond strength to resin cements.[2] Different types of glass ceramics are currently available based on their reinforcement characteristics, and the following materials can be highlighted:

Leucite-reinforced glass-ceramic: This material originates from a glass based on SiO_2, Al_2O_3, and K_2O. The crystallization process via heat treatment causes the growth of leucite crystals ($KAlSi_2O_6$; 35%–45% by volume) in the glassy matrix. Leucite crystals have an important reinforcing effect via the toughening mechanism of crack deflection, resulting in a flexural strength in the range of 160 MPa (IPS Empress CAD, Ivoclar Vivadent, Liechtenstein).[3] The combination of a significant amount of both vitreous phase and crystal reinforcement results in a material that is indicated for restorations in areas with high esthetic demand and moderate occlusal stress, such as veneer restorations and anterior crowns (**Fig. 1**). These glass-ceramics are also available as CAD–CAM blocks with a color gradient for better esthetic results. The material is also available in different translucencies (high and low), increasing the possibilities of mimicking the adjacent tooth structure and also improving the masking ability in cases of discolored substrates by means of reduced light transmission through the LT restorative material.

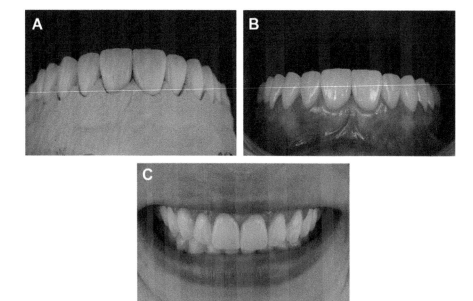

Fig. 1. (*A–C*) Color-gradient leucite reinforced glass-ceramic used for maxillary monolithic restorations. (*Courtesy of* Dr. Manuel Radaelli, Brazil.)

Lithium-disilicate reinforced glass-ceramic: This glass-ceramic is composed essentially of a vitreous phase reinforced by approximately 65% by volume of lithium disilicate crystals, which results in significant reinforcement and leads to a biaxial flexural strength of approximately 450 to 550 MPa (IPS e.max CAD, Ivoclar Vivadent, Liechtenstein).[4] This material is well known for being very versatile and recommended for multiple clinical applications in areas of both occlusal stress and esthetic demand, such as veneers, partial posterior coverages, and anterior and posterior full crowns. Lithium disilicate glass-ceramics are commercially available as CAD–CAM blocks or ingots for the hot-pressing processing method. Both blocks and ingots are available in high, medium, or low translucencies and medium opacity; ingots are also available in high opacity (HO) for the production of copings in cases of severely discolored substrates. The injectable ingots are currently available with a color gradient. This material might be veneered with porcelain (**Fig. 2**) or used in the monolithic form (**Fig. 3**).

Zirconia-reinforced lithium silicate glass-ceramic: The material consists of a glassy matrix composed of lithium metasilicates and lithium orthophosphates. After the crystallization process, particles of lithium silicate are generated. The reinforcement of the vitreous matrix is also provided by the addition of particles of zirconium dioxide ($\sim$10 wt%). This combination creates a material with a biaxial flexural strength of around 540 MPa (Vita Suprinity, Vita Zahnfabrik, and Bad Säckingen, Germany).[5] The reinforcement of the glassy phase makes the material useful for anterior and posterior full crowns, partial occlusal coverages, and veneer restorations. The material is available as CAD–CAM blocks, in the translucent and HT versions.

POLYCRYSTALLINE CERAMICS

This group is represented by materials composed only of a crystalline phase, in the form of crystal grains with no glassy phase. Although alumina has in the past been used frequently in the dental field, zirconia-based ceramics currently dominate this

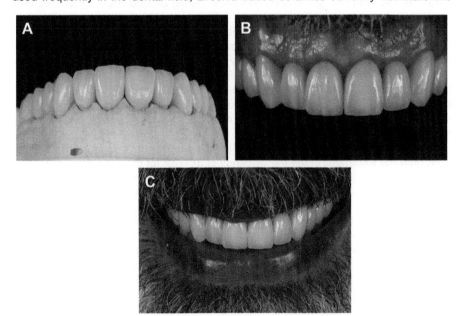

Fig. 2. (*A–C*) Lithium disilicate reinforced glass-ceramic veneered with porcelain—the cutback technique. (*Courtesy of* Dr. Manuel Radaelli, Brazil.)

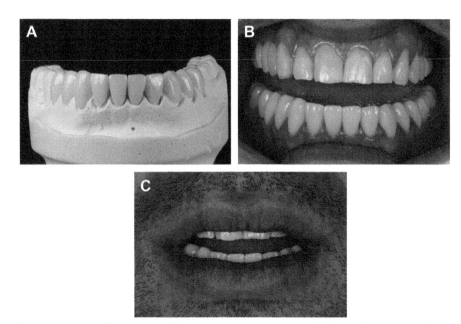

Fig. 3. (*A–C*) Mandibular monolithic restorations are made of lithium disilicate reinforced glass-ceramic. (*Courtesy of* Dr. Manuel Radaelli, Brazil.)

market. Polycrystalline ceramics display high strength, but have low translucency and limited adhesive bonding ability. Over the past decade, dental zirconia has undergone several modifications in its composition in an attempt to equilibrate the so-called 'trade-off' between strength and translucency. Dental zirconia might be divided into two main subgroups:

High-strength polycrystalline ceramics: These materials are composed of zirconium dioxide stabilized in a tetragonal phase by a low volume of yttria (3% mol or 4–6 wt%; 3Y-Tetragonal Zirconial Polycrystal [TZP]).[6] They also have a limited volume of cubic phase in their composition (<15%), and the grain size varies from 0.2 to 1 μm.[6] This class of material has relatively high flexural strength (900–1300 MPa) but also HO.[6] Therefore, its clinical indication ranges from framework structures for single crowns up to multi-unit restorations. The material is commercially available as partially sintered blocks to be milled in a CAD–CAM system.

Translucent polycrystalline ceramics: These materials have been developed to overcome the limitations in the translucency of 3Y-TZP for the production of monolithic restorations (**Fig. 4**). Also, porcelain chipping over zirconia frameworks has been reported as a problem that can be solved with monolithic zirconia restorations. To produce zirconia restorations with higher translucency, an increase in the content of the cubic phase (>15% or > 50%) was necessary, and as a consequence, the level of yttria also need to be increased to 4 or 5 mol%.[6] The resulting materials are the partially stabilized zirconia (PSZ), so-called 4Y-PSZ and 5Y-PSZ. An increase in grain size was also obtained in these materials by raising the sintering temperature. PSZs have been indicated for single and multi-unit monolithic restorations in the anterior and posterior regions (with limitations depending on the manufacturer) with flexural strength ranging from 400 to 1000 MPa.[6] These materials are available in blocks for CAD–CAM milling as monochromatic and, more

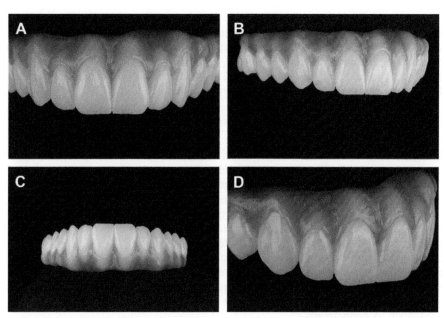

Fig. 4. (*A–D*) Color-gradient and strength-graded translucent zirconia in a full-arch implant-supported restoration. Teeth in monolithic zirconia and porcelain veneering in the gingiva. (*Courtesy of* DT. Marlon Konzen, Brazil.)

recently, with a color-gradient (multi-layer), to improve the optical appearance and characterization, as well as to produce strength-graded structures.

Recent advances in polycrystalline ceramics: New processing methods have been developed to overcome important drawbacks of ceramic restorations. As an example, the veneering of zirconia copings with reinforced glass-ceramic was introduced to reduce the chipping of the veneering layer. In this case, lithium disilicate structures are bonded to zirconia copings through the application of a fusion glass-ceramic (IPS e.max CAD crystall/connect, Ivoclar Vivadent, Liechtenstein). This processing method is called the CAD-on technique. Advances have also occurred in the materials' composition. Manufacturers have developed graded materials combining the high strength of 3Y-TZP with the high translucency of 5Y-PSZ in the same CAD–CAM block (IPS e.max ZIRCAD PRIME, Ivoclar Vivadent, Liechtenstein). This graded material is also available in a color gradient. New technologies for ceramic processing involve alternatives to milling. Stereolithography additive manufacturing (three-dimensional [3D] printing) of zirconia structures has been introduced in the literature and is a promising method due to the possibility of producing structures of more complex geometries and precisely graded properties.[7,8] Examples of zirconia pastes for additive manufacturing include 3DMix ZrO$_2$ paste (3DCeram Co, Limoges, France) and Litha-Con 3Y 210 or 230 (Lithoz, Vienna, Austria). Examples of 3D printers for zirconia are CeraMaker 900 (3DCeram) and CeraFab 7500 Dental (Lithoz).

POLYMER-INFILTRATED CERAMIC NETWORKS

These materials are essentially composed of a partially sintered ceramic matrix (86 wt %) infiltrated with a polymer matrix (14 wt%), and have been developed to combine the advantages of polymeric materials, such as elastic modulus more compatible with that of dentin, with the esthetic outcome and chemical stability of dental ceramics. This combination resulted in flexural strength of approximately 150 MPa (Vita Enamic, Vita Zahnfabrik, Bad Säckingen, Germany).[9] This material is therefore indicated for anterior and posterior crowns, partial occlusal coverage and veneer restorations. It is commercially available as CAD–CAM blocks, with color-gradients or different translucencies depending on the manufacturer.

Essential Properties of Current Dental Ceramics

Strength

Studies have evaluated the strength of ceramics based on the composition or processing technique (**Table 1**). Based on composition, the fatigue performance, referring to fatigue failure loads and survival probabilities, of translucent zirconia has been shown to be superior to that of reinforced glass-ceramics (based on lithium silicate).[10,11] The type of glass-ceramic reinforcement also affects the strength of the material, as zirconia-reinforced lithium silicate had an improved fatigue performance when compared with lithium disilicate for single crowns.[10] The biaxial flexural strength of leucite-reinforced glass-ceramic has been shown to be lower than that obtained with lithium disilicate.[12] PICNs showed lower mechanical performance in comparison to lithium-disilicate reinforced glass-ceramics at traditional thicknesses (~ 1.5 mm),[13-15] but showed similar fatigue performance when used as thicker structures, such as endocrowns.[16]

The fracture strength obtained with the CAD-on technique was similar to that of monolithic translucent zirconia (4Y-PSZ), and both were significantly superior to the strength obtained for monolithic lithium disilicate glass-ceramic or zirconia (high strength) frameworks veneered with porcelain.[17] The same results were observed in regards to survival rates under fatigue loads.[18]

The strength-graded (3Y-TZP/5Y-TZP) monolithic zirconia has shown a higher fracture load than monolithic 4Y-PSZ when evaluated as single crowns after being aged in a chewing simulator.[19]

Regarding the effects of the processing method, previous studies have shown improved fatigue performance[20] and fracture toughness[21] for the pressed technique compared with CAD–CAM processing for lithium disilicate restorations. These differences might be based on the materials' composition, as a higher amount of glassy matrix, reduced crystal phase and smaller crystal size have been observed in IPS e.max CAD.[21] Therefore, this suggests that the crystals' characteristics of IPS e.max Press are more likely to impair crack propagation.[21]

3Y-TZP zirconia structures produced by additive manufacturing (3D printing) have been evaluated. One study showed similar flexural strength for two-printed materials (LithaCon 3Y 230, Lithoz, and 3D Mix zirconia, 3DCeram Sinto) in comparison to a subtractive manufactured (milled) high-strength zirconia (Lava Plus, 3M Oral Care, Seefeld, Germany).[8] However, another study showed lower flexural strength for 3D-printed zirconia (3DMix ZrO2 paste; 3DCeram) in comparison to another milled 3Y-TZP (IPS e.max ZirCAD, Ivoclar Vivadent).[7]

Resistance to wear

Wear of the restorative material or the antagonist has been evaluated in the literature. For the restorative material, a study has shown that lithium disilicate glass-ceramic, feldspathic ceramic, and PICN had greater wear than that of enamel; on the other hand, zirconia structures (3Y-TZP and 5Y-PSZ) showed the lowest wear values, which were significantly lower than that of enamel.[22] Another study has also shown lower volume loss of monolithic zirconia when compared to glass-ceramic (lithium disilicate).[23]

Table 1
Data of studies discussed in the "strength" section, in order as they appear in the text

Authors	Specimen	Properties	Materials	Results
Alves et al.[10]	Simplified crowns	Fatigue failure load (N)	Lithium disilicate (LD) Zirconia-reinforced lithium silicate (ZLS) Translucent zirconia (TZ)	LD = 987[c] ZLS = 1187[b] TZ = 1740[a]
Pereira et al.[11]	Disc-shaped	Fatigue failure load (N)	LD TZ	Dentin analog substrate: LD = 990[b] TZ = 1110[a] Titanium substrate: LD = 1590[b] TZ = 2060[a] Zirconia substrate: LD = 1710[b] TZ = 2300[a]
Lin et al.[12]	Disc shaped	Flexural strength (MPa)	LD Leucite (LC)	1.5 mm thickness: LD = 365.0[a] LC = 163.9[b] 0.8 mm thickness: LD = 367.9[a] LC = 157.6[b]
Mendonça et al.[13]	Crowns	Fracture strength (N)	LD Polymer-infiltrated ceramic network (PICN)	LD = 4100[a] PICN = 2003[b]
Sieper et al.[14]	Crowns	Fracture strength (N) after chewing simulator	LD PICN	1.0 mm thickness LD = 2535[a] PICN = 2128[b] 1.5 mm thickness LD = 2648[a] PICN = 2281[b]
Goujat et al.[15]	Bar shaped	Flexural strength (MPa)	LD PICN	LD = 210.2[a] PICN = 148.7[b]
Dartora et al.[16] 2019	Endocrowns	Fatigue failure load (N)	LD; PICN	LD = 1000[a] PICN = 847[a]

(continued on next page)

Table 1
(continued)

Authors	Specimen	Properties	Materials	Results
Alessandretti et al.[17]	Disc shaped	Fracture load (N)	Zirconia core + LD reinforced glass-ceramic (CAD-on) Zirconia core + porcelain (ZrPc) TZ LD	CAD-on = 3727[a] ZrPc = 3175[b] TZ = 3824[a] LD = 1068[c]
Alessandretti et al.[18] 2020	Disc shaped	Survival time (number of cycles)	Zirconia core + LD reinforced glass-ceramic (CAD-on) Zirconia core + porcelain (ZrPc) TZ LD	CAD-on = 591,071[a] ZrPc = 16,428[c] TZ = 626,785[a] LD = 237,178[b]
Michailova et al.[19]	Crowns	Fracture load (N) after aging	TZ Strength-graded zirconia (SGZ)	TZ (block) = 3949[b] TZ (disc) = 3535[b] SGZ = 5040[a]
Schestatsky et al.[20]	Simplified crowns	Fatigue failure load (N)	Hot-Pressed lithium disilicate (HPLD) Milled lithium disilicate (MLD)	HPLD = 1460[a] MLD = 1200[b]
Alkadi and Ruse[21]	Notchless triangular prism	Fracture toughness (MPa.m$^{1/2}$)	HPLD MLD	HPLD = 2.5[a] MLD = 1.79[b]
Nakai et al.[8]	Bar shaped	Biaxial flexural strength (MPa)	High-strength subtractive zirconia (HSZr) 3D additive Zirconia (Lithacon 3Y 230) 3D additive Zirconia (3D mix zirconia)	HSZr = 1007[ab] Lithacon = 934.8[b] 3D mix = 1071.1[a]
Revilla-León et al.[7]	Bar shaped	Biaxial flexural strength (MPa)	HSZr 3D additive Zirconia	Nonaged HSZr = 914.7[a] 3D = 320.3[b] Aged HSZr = 572.6[a] 3D = 281.1[b]

a,b,c represent the statistical significance among groups.

As for the antagonist, based on *in vitro* analyses, a study has shown lower enamel wear when opposing PICN in comparison to zirconia, lithium disilicate or zirconia-reinforced lithium silicate, which were similar to each other.[24] Another study has also shown greater wear of enamel opposing lithium disilicate in comparison to PICN; and both materials provided greater wear than the enamel–enamel combination.[25] A study showed that zirconia led to lower volume loss of antagonist enamel than glass-ceramics (leucite and lithium disilicate).[26] Regarding monolithic zirconia, studies have shown that a highly polished material is essential to ensure reduced antagonist wear,[27,28] as the surface roughness of zirconia was a predictor of wear of opposing dentition.[27]

Clinical studies compared the wear of enamel tested against monolithic zirconia and glass-ceramics. As shown by a systematic review of in vivo studies, the wear of enamel tested against zirconia was similar to or greater than that observed against natural teeth, but lower than that measured against a glass-ceramic.[29] The same outcome was observed in a more recent clinical study.[30]

Optical properties

Translucency and color differences are two of the main optical properties of dental ceramics for consideration in daily practice. Knowledge about these properties will allow clinicians to choose materials to mimic the translucency of the neighboring structures or to mask discolored substrates. The translucency parameter (TP_{00}) of high-strength polycrystalline ceramics veneered with porcelain or glass-ceramics (CAD-on) has been shown to be significantly lower than those of monolithic glass-ceramics or translucent zirconia.[31] The use of veneered zirconia copings was particularly desirable to be used over severely discolored substrates (such as those with shades of A3.5 or C4, and metallic structures) because they provided adequate masking ability (based on color differences, ΔE_{00}), which was not achieved with monolithic restorations. The CAD-on technique improved the masking ability over metal backgrounds when compared with zirconia coping veneered with porcelain. Considering monolithic structures, leucite-reinforced glass-ceramics and highly translucent lithium disilicate showed higher TP_{00} mean values, which were superior to those obtained for translucent zirconia and low-translucent lithium disilicate, both of which showed similar TP_{00} values.[31] These monolithic structures showed an inability to mask severely discolored backgrounds, as shown by the high color differences measured in previous reports.[31] To overcome this problem, CAD–CAM monolithic ceramic materials need to be associated with opaque luting agents or the application to the preparation of high-value opaque flowable resin composites before the production of the ceramic restoration.[32]

Precision (marginal and internal fit)

Similar results regarding precision have been observed in the literature for a wide range of CAD–CAM processed materials. The mean marginal internal gaps were similar when lithium disilicate was compared with zirconia-reinforced lithium silicate for milled veneers.[33] The marginal fit of zirconia and lithium disilicate crowns did not show significant differences in another report.[33] Marginal and internal fit of lithium disilicate and PICN were similar and lower than 100 μm when evaluated as inlay restorations.[34] Another analysis has shown that monolithic and bilayer CAD–CAM zirconia crowns displayed marginal gaps that were within an acceptable range of clinical discrepancy and statistically similar to each other.[35]

The differences among the processing methods are fairly evident from a review of the literature. One study has shown differences in precision when CAD–CAM and pressed lithium disilicate crowns were compared regarding marginal adaptation, with better results for the latter. However, when internal gaps were considered, milled crowns showed lower values.[36] Differences were also found between leucite-based glass-ceramics and zirconia-reinforced lithium silicate monolithic crowns produced by milling or the pressing technique, with better results for the CAD–CAM method.[37] One study compared the marginal and internal fit of pressed lithium disilicate crowns with wax patterns produced manually, by 3D printing, or milled; the study indicated that better results were obtained with the CAD–CAM subtractive milling method.[38] Another study evaluated the precision of tabletops produced by 3D-printed zirconia, milled zirconia, and pressed lithium disilicate, and showed the milled CAD–CAM technique to be more precise than the hot-pressing method and the 3D-printing technique for most of the measured points.[39] The precision of 3D-printed zirconia crowns was evaluated in comparison with the conventional milling technique.[40] The study showed that the milled group had lower internal and marginal discrepancies compared with the group processed by additive manufacturing. However, all values were below a clinically acceptable range.

SUMMARY

Advances in dental ceramics have been made with the aim of producing materials that are more resistant to wear and fracture, and with improved optical properties to facilitate mimicking the natural dental structures. These aims have been achieved by increasing both the translucency of polycrystalline materials and the strength of the glass-ceramics. The development of color-gradient and strength-graded materials is also remarkable achievements. Also, the production of precise ceramic restorations has been achieved by using technologies such as computer-aided designs (CADs) and milling machines or, more recently, 3D printing. Continued improvements in these directions are likely to increase the predictability of dental treatments based on ceramic restorations.

CLINICS CARE POINTS

- Monolithic restorations of glass ceramics, PICN, or translucent zirconia are adequate in terms of strength, wear, and precision, but must be considered carefully in discolored substrates because of their improved translucency.
- Highly reinforced glass-ceramics or translucent zirconia should be considered with priority for monolithic restorations in patients with high occlusal forces.
- The current fabrication methods such as milling, pressing, or 3D-printing are adequate to provided restorations clinically acceptable in term of fit.

ACKNOWLEDGMENTS

The authors are grateful to Dr Manuel Tomas Borges Radaelli (see **Figs. 1–3**) and DT. Marlon Konzen (see **Fig. 4**) for their generous support with illustrations.

DISCLOSURE

The authors have nothing to disclose.

REFERENCES

1. Moshaverinia A. Review of the modern dental ceramic restorative materials for esthetic dentistry in the minimally invasive age. Dent Clin North Am 2020;64:621–31.

2. Seghi RR, Del Rio DL. Biomaterials: ceramic and adhesive technologies. Dent Clin North Am 2019;63:233–48.
3. Ivoclar vivadent. IPS Empress CAD® Scientific documentation. 2011.
4. Ivoclar vivadent. IPS E.max CAD® Scientific documentation. 2005.
5. Vita zahnfabrik. Vita Suprinity® PC Technical and scientific documentation. 2016.
6. Zhang Y, Lawn BR. Novel zirconia materials in dentistry. J Dent Res 2018;97: 140–7.
7. León MR, Husain NA, Ceballos L, et al. Flexural strength and Weibull characteristics of stereolithography additive manufactured versus milled zirconia. J Prosthet Dent 2021;125:685–90.
8. Nakai H, Inokoshi M, Nozaki K, et al. Additive manufactured zirconia for dental applications. Materials 2021;14:3694.
9. Vita zahnfabrik. Vita Enamic® Technical and scientific documentation. 2013.
10. Alves DM, Cadore-Rodrigues AC, Prochnow C, et al. Fatigue performance of adhesively luted glass or polycrystalline CAD–CAM monolithic crowns. J Prosthet Dent 2021;126:119–27.
11. Pereira GKR, Graunke P, Maroli A, et al. Lithium disilicate glass-ceramic vs translucent zirconia polycrystals bonded to distinct substrates: Fatigue failure load, number of cycles for failure, survival rates, and stress distribution. J Mech Behav Biomed Mater 2019;91:122–30.
12. Lin W, Ercoli C, Feng C, et al. The effect of core material, veneering porcelain, and fabrication technique on the biaxial flexural strength and Weibull analysis of selected dental ceramics. J Prosthodont 2012;21:353–62.
13. Mendonça AF, Shahmoradi M, Gouvêa CVD, et al. Microstructural and mechanical characterization of CAD/CAM materials for monolithic dental restorations. J Prosthodont 2019;28:e587–94.
14. Sieper K, Wille S, Kern M. Fracture strength of lithium disilicate crowns compared to polymer-infiltrated ceramic-network and zirconia reinforced lithium silicate crowns. J Mech Behav Biomed Mater 2017;74:342–8.
15. Goujat A, Abouelleil H, Colon P, et al. Mechanical properties and internal fit of 4 CAD–CAM block materials. J Prosthet Dent 2018;119:384–9.
16. Dartora G, Rocha Pereira GK, Varella de Carvalho R, et al. Comparison of endocrowns made of lithium disilicate glass-ceramic or polymer-infiltrated ceramic networks and direct composite resin restorations: fatigue performance and stress distribution. J Mech Behav Biomed Mater 2019;100:103401.
17. Alessandretti R, Borba M, Benetti P, et al. Reliability and mode of failure of bonded monolithic and multilayer ceramics. Dent Mater 2017;33:191–7.
18. Alessandretti R, Borba M, Della Bona A. Cyclic contact fatigue resistance of ceramics for monolithic and multilayer dental restorations. Dent Mater 2020;36: 535–41.
19. Michailova M, Elsayed A, Fabel G, et al. Comparison between novel strength-gradient and color-gradient multilayer zirconia using conventional and high-speed sintering. J Mech Behav Biomed Mater 2020;111:103977.
20. Schestatsky R, Zucuni CP, Venturini AB, et al. CAD–CAM milled versus pressed lithium-disilicate monolithic crowns adhesively cemented after distinct surface treatments: Fatigue performance and ceramic surface characteristics. J Mech Behav Biomed Mater 2019;94:144–54.
21. Alkadi L, Ruse ND. Fracture toughness of two lithium disilicate dental glass ceramics. J Prosthet Dent 2016;116:591–6.
22. Borrero-Lopez O, Guiberteau F, Zhang Y, et al. Wear of ceramic-based dental materials. J Mech Behav Biomed Mater 2019;92:144–51.

23. Zurek AD, Alfro MF, Wee AG, et al. Wear characteristics and volume loss of CAD/CAM ceramic materials. J Prosthotont 2019;28:e510–8.

24. Ludovichetti FS, Trindade FZ, Werner A, et al. Wear resistance and abrasiveness of CAD–CAM monolithic materials. J Prosthet Dent 2018;120:318.e1–8.

25. Lawson NC, Bansal R, Burgess JO. Wear, strength, modulus and hardness of CAD/CAM restorative materials. Dent Mater 2016;31:e275–83.

26. Nakashima J, Taira Y, Sawase T. In vitro wear of four ceramic materials and human enamel on enamel antagonist. Eur J Oral Sci 2016;124:295–300.

27. Janyavula S, Lawson NC, Cakir D, et al. The wear of polished and glazed zirconia against enamel. J Prosthet Dent 2013;109:22–9.

28. Matzinger M, Hahnel S, Preis V, et al. Polishing effects and wear performance of chairside CAD/CAM materials. Clin Oral Investig 2019;23:725–37.

29. Gou M, Chen H, Kang J, et al. Antagonist enamel wear of tooth-supported monolithic zirconia posterior crowns in vivo: A systematic review. J Prosthet Dent 2019;121:598–603.

30. Deval P, Tembhurne J, Gangurde A, et al. A clinical comparative evaluation of the wear of enamel antagonist to monolithic zirconia and metal-ceramic crowns. Int J Prosthodont 2021;34:744–51.

31. Bacchi A, Boccardi S, Alessandretti R, et al. Substrate masking ability of bilayer and monolithic ceramics used for complete crowns and the effect of association with an opaque resin-based luting agent. J Prosthodont Res 2019;63:321–6.

32. Dotto L, Soares PM, Slongo S, et al. Layering of discolored substrates with high-value opaque composites for CAD–CAM monolithic ceramics. J Prosthet Dent 2021;126:128.e1–6.

33. Baig MR, Akbar AA, Sabti MY, et al. Evaluation of marginal and internal fit of a CAD/CAM monolithic zirconia-reinforced lithium silicate porcelain laminate veneer system. J Prosthodont 2021.

34. Uzgur R, Ercan E, Uzgur Z, et al. Cement thickness of inlay restorations made of lithium disilicate, polymer-infiltrated ceramic and nano-ceramic CAD/CAM materials evaluated using 3D X-ray micro-computed tomography. J Prothodont 2018;27:456–60.

35. Piñal MD, Lopez-Suarez C, Bartolome JF, et al. Effect of cementation and aging on the marginal fit of veneered and monolithic zirconia and metal-ceramic CAD–CAM crowns. J Prosthet Dent 2021;125:323.e1–7.

36. Schestatsky R, Zucuni CP, Dapieve KS, et al. Microstructure, topography, surface roughness, fractal dimension, internal and marginal adaptation of pressed and milled lithium-disilicate monolithic restorations. J Prosthodont Res 2020;64:12–9.

37. Vasiliu RD, Porojan SD, Porojan L. In vitro study of comparative evaluation of marginal and internal fit between heat-pressed and CAD–CAM monolithic glass-ceramic restorations after thermal aging. Materials 2020;13(19):4239.

38. Homsy FR, Özcan M, Khoury M, et al. Marginal and internal fit of pressed and lithium disilicate inlays fabricated with milling, 3D printing, and conventional technologies. J Prosthet Dent 2018;119:783–90.

39. Loannidis A, Park JM, Hüsler J, et al. An in vitro comparison of the marginal and internal adaptation of ultrathin occlusal veneers made of 3D-printed zirconia, milled zirconia, and heat-pressed lithium disilicate. J Prosthet Dent 2021;S0022-3913(20):30722–8.

40. Revilla-León M, Methani MM, Morton D, et al. Internal and marginal discrepancies associated with stereolithography (SLA) additive manufactured zirconia crowns. J Prosthet Dent 2020;124:730–7.

Current Protocols for Resin-Bonded Dental Ceramics

Markus B. Blatz, DMD, PhD[a],*, Julian Conejo, DMD, MSc[a], Amirah Alammar, BDS[b], Jose Ayub, DDS[a]

KEYWORDS

- Ceramics • Resin bonding • Surface treatment • Resin cements • Longevity

KEY POINTS

- Clinical outcomes of resin-bonded dental ceramics depend on the type and microstructure of the ceramic and the respective adhesive protocol.
- Understanding the composition and microstructure of dental ceramics is critical for selecting the proper resin-bonding protocol: successful methods differ significantly for silica-based and metal-oxide ceramics.
- Long-term durable adhesion to dental ceramics relies on a dual bond: micromechanical interlocking and true chemical bonds to the substrate.
- Surface pretreatment methods create a surface topography that facilitates micromechanical interlocking and decontaminate the bonding substrate.
- Material-dependent priming and bonding agents form chemical bonds to the ceramic.

INTRODUCTION

Clinical success of resin-bonded ceramic restorations is influenced by the ceramic material physical and optical properties, tooth preparation design, impression technique, fabrication process, and definitive insertion protocol.[1,2] Proper bonding protocols facilitate adhesion of the restorative material to the tooth,[3] enhance marginal adaptation,[4] prevent microleakage,[5] and increase fracture resistance of the prepared tooth and the restoration itself.[6] There are two distinctly different interfaces to consider: the one to the tooth and the other one to the restorative material. The ideal bonding protocol should provide a dual bond: micromechanical interlocking and true chemical bonds to various types of dental ceramics.[7–9] Micromechanical interlocking is created through infiltration of priming agents, silane coupling agents, and cements into microretentive bonding surfaces. In addition, resin cements should have

[a] Department of Preventive and Restorative Sciences, University of Pennsylvania School of Dental Medicine, 240 South 40th Street, Philadelphia, PA 19104, USA; [b] Sijam Medical Center, Northern Ring Road, Alghadeer District, Riyadh, Saudi Arabia
* Corresponding author.
E-mail address: mblatz@upenn.edu

Dent Clin N Am 66 (2022) 603–625
https://doi.org/10.1016/j.cden.2022.05.008
0011-8532/22/© 2022 Elsevier Inc. All rights reserved.

dental.theclinics.com

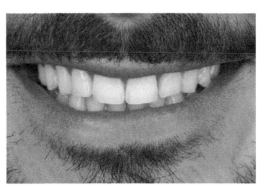

Fig. 1. Preoperative extraoral view.

physiochemical properties similar to tooth structure, biocompatibility, resistance to solubility, and chemical and color stability.[10–12]

The composition of the resin cement and the pretreatment methods applied to restorative material and tooth surfaces greatly influences the longevity of bonded ceramic restorations.[5] Surface pretreatment is defined as one or a series of steps to enhance the surface topography on a microscopic level: acid etching, mechanical roughening, cleaning, and removal of any debris and contaminants.[13]

Resin cements are typically a composition of bis-GMA or urethane dimethacrylate resin matrix and 20% to 80% inorganic filler particles.[14] They are often classified as resin-modified glass ionomer and composite resin cements, which is further classified according to their activation mode: light-activated, dual-activated, and autoactivated.[15] Other classification systems distinguish between bonding techniques, which either require pretreatment steps (total and self-etch adhesive systems) or without any pretreatment steps to the bonded tooth surface (self-adhesive systems).[16] Each of them have different indications, which makes their proper selection challenging.[17]

There are several types of surface pretreatment methods that are applied to dental ceramics. The most common ones are etching with hydrofluoric acid (HF), airborne-particle abrasion (APA) with aluminum oxide or glass beads, tribochemical silica coating (TBS), and lasers.[5,18–20] Selection of the proper treatment is dictated by type, composition, and mechanical properties of the specific ceramic. The nature and microstructure of the ceramic determines its strength and optical properties.

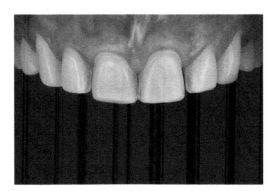

Fig. 2. Veneer preparations from maxillary left first premolar to right first premolar.

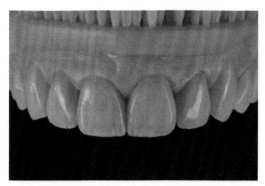

Fig. 3. Silica-based ceramic laminate veneers on printed model.

Early mentioning of ceramics applied in dentistry date back to the eighteenth century, when Alexis Duchateau fabricated complete dentures using porcelain.[21] This innovation led to further exploration of different applications of ceramics as a restorative material. In the late 1800s, Richmond fabricated a porcelain single-piece crown fused to a metal post,[22] which was followed by the development of all-porcelain jacket crowns by Charles Land in 1889.[23] These crowns had excellent esthetics but their low mechanical strength resulted in a high incidence of clinical failures.[24] Further developments increased their strength and toughness.[25]

Today, ceramics are classified by their microstructure into silica-based ceramics, resin-matrix ceramics, and oxide ceramics.[26] Advancements in fabrication processes and digital technologies expanded their clinical applications to inlays,[27,28] onlays,[29,30] veneers,[31,32] resin-bonded prostheses,[33,34] copings,[35,36] crowns,[37,38] short- and long-span fixed dental prostheses,[39,40] and implant components and implant-supported fixed dental prostheses.[41,42] Bonding to brittle silica-based ceramics is highly predictable because of their high glass content.[5,43] However, the composition and physical properties of oxide ceramics require fundamentally different bonding protocols to achieve strong and long-term durable resin bonds.[18,44]

BONDING TO SILICA-BASED CERAMICS

Silica-based ceramics are nonmetallic inorganic amorphous materials that contain a glass phase. They are divided into traditional feldspathic ceramics, leucite-

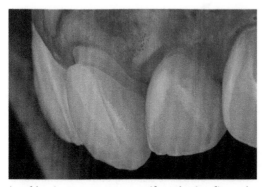

Fig. 4. Intraoral try-in of laminate veneers to verify esthetics, fit, and occlusion.

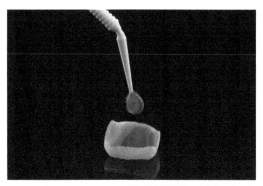

Fig. 5. Laminate veneer surface treatment with 9.8% HF acid for 2 minutes.

reinforced glass ceramics, and lithium silicate ceramics.[45] The glass phase offers high translucency, excellent esthetics, and a natural appearance.[46] Their brittleness and low mechanical properties require adhesive bonding.[47] Durable bonds to silica-based ceramics are best established through HF acid etching followed by application of a silane coupling agent.[5] The etching time and concentration of the etchant depend on the amount of glass and crystalline content of the ceramic.[9]

BONDING TO TRADITIONAL FELDSPATHIC CERAMICS

Feldspathic ceramics are a mixture of leucite (potassium aluminosilicate) and glass. They have low to medium values of flexural strength up to 120 MPa[48] and are considered the most translucent and esthetic ceramic materials. They are typically used as veneering material for metal or ceramic copings and frameworks; bonded laminate veneers; inlays/onlays; and even full-coverage crowns, especially the ones fabricated with chairside computer-aided design/computer-aided manufacturing (CAD/CAM) technology. However, because of their low flexural strength, they are not recommended for patients with severe bruxism or for use in areas with high occlusal load.[49]

A 95.5% survival rate after up to 10 years was reported for bonded feldspathic veneers.[50] Inlays and onlays showed a survival rate probability of 88.7% after up to 17 years of clinical service.[51] Of the 11% failures, no debonding incidences were reported.

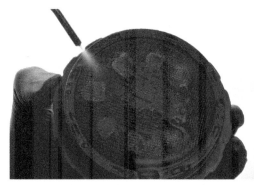

Fig. 6. Cleaning of veneers in ultrasonic cleaning bath in alcohol for 5 minutes to remove debris and remnants from acid etching.

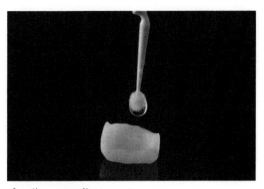

Fig. 7. Application of a silane coupling agent.

Feldspathic ceramic surfaces undergo dissolution when exposed to HF acid, which selectively dissolves its glass phase, exposing silicon dioxide and yielding to topographic changes in the surface that contribute to micromechanical interlocking and chemical bonds with a silane and resin cements.[52] HF creates a roughened surface, thus increasing the wettability of the ceramic surface and modifying internal surface flaws present within the ceramic surface.[53,54] It also cleans and decontaminates the bonding surfaces by removing unwanted oxides, phosphates, and other contaminants that cover the surface during manufacturing and try-in procedures. The effect of the acid etchant depends on its concentration and the etching time.[55] Higher HF concentrations may weaken the ceramic surface[53] and significantly lower flexural strength was found when acid concentrations were increased.[56] Conversely, higher concentrations of HF acid produced more intense topographic surface changes of the feldspathic ceramics, facilitating better mechanical interlocking with resin cements.[9] A more uniform crystal structure was observed as a result of the dissolved glass phase with high HF acid concentrations than with lower concentrations and stable long-term resin bonds were achieved.[57] For feldspathic ceramics, 9.8% HF acid applied for 2 minutes is recommended, followed by silane application.[45]

Light-cure resin cements are used for feldspathic veneers to provide extended working times and simplified removal of cement excess before light-activation, which reduces time for finishing and polishing after bonding.[58,59] In addition, light-cure composite resins have a good color stability because they do not contain chemical

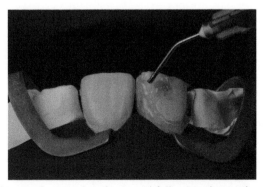

Fig. 8. Enamel etching with 35% phosphoric acid following the total etch technique.

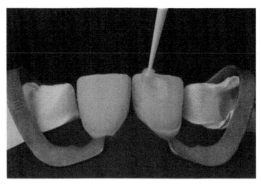

Fig. 9. Bonding agent application.

activators, such as tertiary amines, which may cause color changes in the long term.[10,60] Dual-cure resin cements combine the advantages of light- and chemical-activated resin cements.[61] They reach adequate degrees of polymerization and provide an extended working time because of the controlled light-activation mechanism.[62] They have the highest mechanical properties and hardness compared with other activation mechanisms. However, dual-cure resin cements may have reduced color stability, because of possible oxidation of the tertiary amines.[63,64] They are recommended for bonding of feldspathic inlays/onlays and in clinical situations where the light from the curing unit cannot reach all regions of the cavity or deep internal areas of the preparation.[65] Furthermore, different bonding protocols (total-etch, self-etch, and self-adhesive resin cements) showed similar results in the long term.[66] However, total-etch systems form a strong bonding interface between the tooth and the ceramic surface and reduce microleakage around feldspathic veneers better than self-etch systems.[67]

BONDING TO LEUCITE-REINFORCED GLASS CERAMICS

With an increased strength over traditional feldspathic ceramics, leucite-reinforced feldspathic ceramics are indicated for anterior crowns, inlays, and onlays.[45] They contain up to 45% by volume of leucite,[68] which is a reinforcing phase that results in medium flexural strength values of up to 140 MPa and acts as a crack reflector that contributes to the increased resistance to crack propagation.[48]

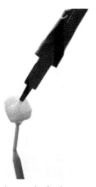

Fig. 10. Application of light-cure composite resin luting agent.

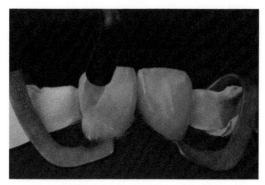

Fig. 11. Removal of excess cement before light curing for 20 seconds from each side.

A 94.6% survival rate was found for leucite-reinforced ceramic inlays and onlays after up to 5 years.[69] Leucite-reinforced feldspathic ceramic crowns showed high survival rates of 95.2.% and excellent esthetics after up to 11 years.[70] None of the failed restorations experienced loss of retention. Because of their lower glass phase compared with conventional feldspathic ceramics, 9.8% HF acid etching for 1 minute is recommend.[45] Various types of resin cements showed similar long-term outcomes, as long as HF acid–etched surfaces were silanated.[66,71,72]

BONDING TO LITHIUM SILICATE CERAMICS

Lithium silicate ceramics became popular because of their esthetic properties and greater flexural strength than leucite-reinforced ceramics.[73] They are heat pressed or CAD/CAM fabricated with a glass phase consisting of lithium disilicate and lithium orthophosphate, which increases fracture resistance without negatively influencing translucency.[45] With a flexural strength of up to 470 MPa, they are the strongest silica-based ceramic.[26]

Lithium silicate ceramics are used for inlays, onlays, crowns, three-unit fixed dental prosthesis in the anterior region, and implant-supported crowns.[45,74] Survival rates of 96.7% and 95.2% were reported for pressed lithium silicate posterior full coverage crowns and partial coverage inlays and onlays.[75] No debonding incidences were observed during the 16.9 years clinical follow-up. Short- and medium-term survival rates are also high[76,77] with clinically acceptable fracture strength values.[30]

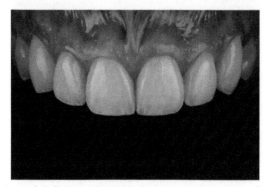

Fig. 12. Intraoral view of definitive silica-based ceramic restorations after bonding.

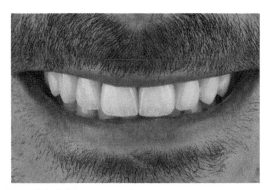

Fig. 13. Extraoral view of definitive restorations.

As with all silica-based ceramics, HF acid etch is recommend for roughening the lithium silicate surface for durable resin bonds.[78] Because HF etching removes the glass phase between the crystals, lithium silicate ceramics require only 20 seconds of etching with a lower HF acid concentration of 4.6%, followed by an application of a silane coupling agent.[45] Various resin cements showed durable resin bonds in the long term.[75,79–81] To simplify bonding protocols and decrease technique sensitivity, manufacturers have recently developed universal bonding agents, which are not only indicated to bond to tooth structures but also to a large variety of dental materials. They typically contain a silane to expand their range of indications to silica-based ceramics. However, their specific concentration and the impact of other components on the reactivity of the silane within this "mix" seems to make them less effective, urging researchers to recommend a separate layer of silane to optimize bond strengths.[82]

These findings apply to all silica-based ceramics.[83] It should also be noted that several recently developed "ceramic primers" contain a silane and special phosphate monomers, making them applicable to silica-based and metal-oxide ceramics.

The clinical treatment steps involved in successful resin bonding of silica-based ceramics previously detailed are illustrated with a clinical case, depicted in **Figs. 1–13**.

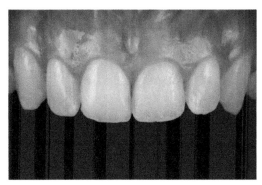

Fig. 14. Intraoral preoperative situation. Maxillary right central incisor required full coverage restoration.

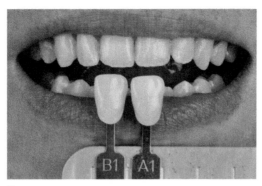

Fig. 15. Shade selection.

BONDING TO POLYMER-INFILTRATED CERAMIC NETWORK MATERIALS

Polymer-infiltrated ceramic network (PICN) materials seek to combine the advantages of ceramics and polymers. They consist of interpenetrating networks of ceramic and polymer, with an aluminum oxide–enriched, fine structured leucite (86 wt%), into which 14% wt urethane dimethacrylate and triethylene glycol dimethacrylate polymer material is injected[84] to imitate the mechanical behavior of natural teeth.[85,86] They offer reduced brittleness and rigidity, improved flexibility and fracture toughness, and better machinability than silica-based ceramics.[87] Although milling times are reduced, they provide better internal and marginal accuracy with simplified finishing procedures.[88] Similar to composite materials, abrasive wear of opposing teeth is low.[89,90] When applied for resin-bonded restorative treatment options, APA with alumina particles, phosphoric acid, and HF acid etch have been suggested as surface pretreatment methods.[84,91,92] A systematic review on bonding to PICN concluded that APA with alumina followed by silane application was the most feasible method.[93] However, recent studies report that 5% HF etching for 1 minute followed by silanization is the best bonding protocol.[84,87,93] After etching with HF acid, the surface topography is characterized by the exposure of the polymer network as the ceramic matrix is selectively removed.[94] Furthermore, the methoxy groups present in the silane chemically bond with ceramics and integrated polymer components, polymerizing with the

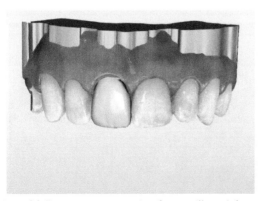

Fig. 16. Digital design of full-coverage restoration for maxillary right central incisor.

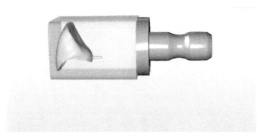

Fig. 17. A high-translucent zirconia crown was milled with chairside CAD/CAM system.

methacrylate groups of the resin cements.[95] Various types of resin cements showed similar bond strength values.[84,93]

BONDING TO METAL-OXIDE CERAMICS

When categorized by microstructure, oxide ceramics are non-glass-based systems. Their fine-grain crystalline structure provides strength and toughness with limited translucency.[74] In addition, the absence of the glass phase limits the effectiveness of HF acid etching, requiring alternative surface pretreatment methods to the ones applied to silica-based and PICN materials.[18]

Oxide ceramics, such as alumina and zirconia, are typically fabricated with CAD/CAM technologies and were developed as alternatives to porcelain-fused-to-metal restorations.[43] Yttria-stabilized zirconium dioxide ceramics (Y-TZP) have gained popularity in daily dental practice, first as coping and framework materials to be veneered with layering porcelain and more recently to fabricate full-contour monolithic restorations.[96,97] The yttria content in zirconia largely defines its mechanical and optical properties. Different generations of zirconia are classified according to their yttria content into 3Y-TZP, 4Y-TZP, and 5Y-TZP,[98,99] each of them having specific mechanical properties, optical properties, and, consequently, clinical indications. One of the great advantages of oxide-based versus silica-based ceramics is that they do not

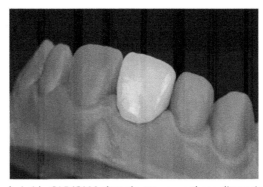

Fig. 18. Definitive chairside CAD/CAM zirconia crown on three-dimensional printed model.

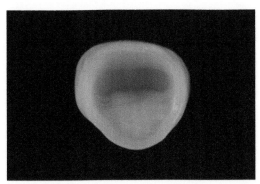

Fig. 19. Full-coverage zirconia crowns do not require resin bonding and is cemented conventionally. However, resin bonding increases flexural strength, especially for thin high-translucent zirconia crowns, which are more translucent but weaker than the ones made from conventional zirconia.

require resin bonding for definitive insertion of full-coverage restorations. They are conventionally cemented as long as restoration retention and fit are adequate.[5]

3Y-TZP is partially stabilized in the tetragonal phase and has the highest fracture toughness and flexural strength (>1000 MPa) among zirconia generations.[100–102] They are indicated as a coping and framework structure for all bilayer all-ceramic crowns, resin-bonded prosthesis, fixed partial dentures, implant abutments, endodontic posts, tooth and implant supported frameworks, overdenture bars, and full mouth reconstructions.[43] Properties termed "active crack resistance" or "transformation toughening" are unique to this material, because it undergoes tetragonal-to-monoclinic phase transformation that limits crack propagation, enhancing its fracture toughness and flexural strength.[103,104]

Several surface pretreatment methods have been found to improve resin bonds to 3Y-TZP, such as APA with aluminum oxide or glass beads, TBS, low-fusion porcelain application, hot chemical etching solutions, selective infiltration etching, laser irradiation, plasma spraying, and zirconia ceramic powder coating.[43,105,106] In vitro studies dating back to the early 2000s and systematic reviews are in strong agreement that a combination of mechanical and chemical pretreatment is necessary for long-term

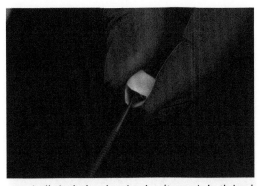

Fig. 20. The first step typically includes cleaning in ultrasonic bath in alcohol. Alternatively, novel zirconia cleaning agents can successfully decontaminate bonding surfaces (shown here: Katana Cleaner, Kuraray Noritake, Tokyo, Japan).

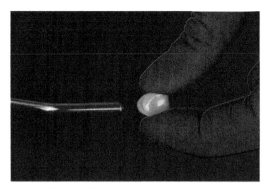

Fig. 21. Zirconia cleaner is rinsed off and restoration is dried.

durable resin bonds to 3Y-TZP.[16,43,107,108] Application of 10-methacryloyloxydecyl dihydrogen phosphate (MDP) monomer or phosphate ester monomer-based primers and resin cements on surface-treated 3Y-TZP provide superior and long-term durable resin bonds.[109,110] These functional monomers bond chemically to the metal-oxides in Y-TZP.[18]

The preferred bonding protocol to 3Y-TZP has three key steps, summarized in the widely known APC zirconia bonding concept: APA with alumina or silica-coated alumina particles (step A), priming of the air-abraded surfaces with an MDP or phosphate-monomer-based primer (step P), and a dual or self-cure composite resin cement (step C).[111]

Systematic reviews have also assessed in vitro and clinical durability of different bonding protocols for 3Y-TZP to enamel, dentin, composite cores, titanium abutments and bases, zirconia abutments, and lithium disilicate crowns.[16,112] They come to the same conclusion that APA in combination with MDP monomer-based primer and/or resin cements provide superior and long-term durable bond strengths. Air abrasion with small alumina- or silica-coated particles (50–60 μm) at low pressure (2 bar) was found to be sufficient.[45]

High-translucent 4Y-TZP and 5Y-TZP are more recent generations of zirconia. Enhanced esthetics by increasing the yttria content to 4% and 5% mol makes them applicable for full-contour monolithic restorations, without the need for an additional veneering ceramic layer.[113] The increased yttria content results in a higher percentage

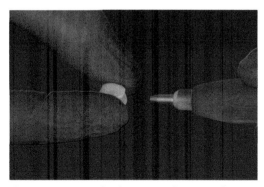

Fig. 22. APC protocol step A: air-particle abrasion with 50-μm aluminum oxide.

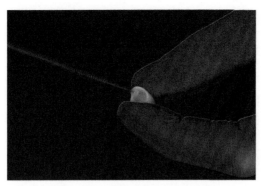

Fig. 23. APC protocol step P: special zirconia primer application.

of cubic-phase particles, which make those compositions more translucent and less susceptible to low temperature degradation than 3Y-TZP.[102,114] Transformation toughening, one of the key factor for superior flexural strength, does not occur with these compositions. Consequently, their reduced flexural strength and fracture toughness limits their clinical indications to single-unit and short-span fixed partial denture restorations.[115–117] Concerns were raised regarding surface pretreatment methods applied to those more recent zirconia generations and their impact on flexural strength.[103,118] These methods include APA with alumina or glass beads,[119–121] TBS,[122,123] plasma treatment,[124] and piranha and hot chemical etching solutions.[125]

A systematic review on bonding to new generations of zirconia found no negative effect of surface pretreatment methods on flexural strength.[126] Bonding protocols applied to 3Y-TZP zirconia are also successful for 4Y-TZP and 5Y-TZP zirconia. Combining mechanical surface pretreatment methods with special phosphate monomer-containing primers and/or composite resin cements provides durable resin bonds. APA with small alumina particles (50 μm) at low pressure (2 bar) is recommended.[101]

Several recently developed "ceramic primers" contain a silane and special phosphate monomers, such as MDP (eg, Clearfil Ceramic Primer Plus, Kuraray Noritake Dental, Tokyo, Japan), making them applicable and effective to silica-based and Y-TZP ceramics. Some authors recommend APA with glass beads. Here, application of a combined silane-MDP primer provides the highest bond strengths.[127]

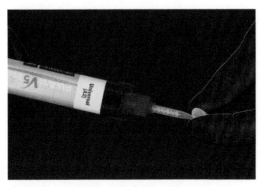

Fig. 24. APC protocol step C: composite resin luting agent.

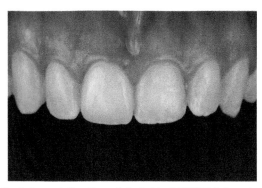

Fig. 25. Postoperative intraoral situation of chairside CAD/CAM zirconia crown on maxillary right central incisor.

One of the advantages of using zirconia is that full-coverage crowns with adequate thickness and retention do not require resin bonding and is cemented conventionally. However, in some clinical situations, resin bonding may be indicated to increase retention and flexural strength, especially for the weaker high-translucent zirconia options. The clinical steps applied in such situation are depicted in **Figs. 14–27**.

Proper isolation during resin-bonding procedures is critical to avoid contamination, which could potentially compromise clinical success. Application of rubber dam and use of gauze pieces, cotton rolls, Teflon tape, gingival retraction cords, and proper suction devices[128,129] may limit contamination with moisture, bacteria, saliva, and blood to improve the quality and longevity of the bonded ceramic restorations.[128]

Alcohol solutions, such as ethanol and isopropanol, and phosphoric acid can clean ceramic surfaces after intraoral restoration try-in procedures.[100] Phosphoric acid for 1 minute and ultrasonic cleaning for 5 minutes were recommended for cleaning silica-based ceramics before application of silane coupling agents.[87] APA with alumina particles was found to be a more effective decontamination and cleaning method for oxide ceramics than alcohol solutions.[112] Recontamination after cleaning occurs even when the restoration is only exposed to air, leading to lower bond strength values to zirconia when more time elapses between APA and primer application.[130] Still, many clinicians, especially the ones who do not have access to a sandblasting unit or microetcher, prefer to have the dental laboratory conduct the APA of

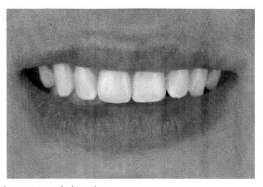

Fig. 26. Postoperative extraoral situation.

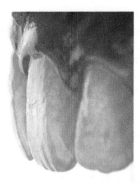

Fig. 27. Postoperative lateral view.

Table 1
Recommended bonding protocols for ceramic restorations

Ceramic	Bonding Protocol
Traditional feldspathic ceramics	1. Intraoral restoration try-in 2. Etch with 9.8% HF acid for 2 min, rinse, and dry 3. Ultrasonic cleaning in alcohol for 5 min 4. Silane application for 20 s and dry 5. Proper isolation 6. Pretreat tooth surfaces 7. Light-cure or dual-cure composite resin luting agent
Leucite-reinforced glass ceramics	1. Intraoral restoration try-in 2. Etch with 9.8% HF acid for 1 min, rinse, and dry 3. Ultrasonic cleaning in alcohol for 5 min 4. Silane application for 20 s and dry 5. Proper isolation 6. Pretreat tooth surfaces 7. Light-cure or dual-cure composite resin luting agent
Lithium silicate ceramics	1. Intraoral restoration try-in 2. Etch with 4.6% HF acid for 20 s, rinse, and dry 3. Ultrasonic cleaning in alcohol for 5 min 4. Silane application for 20 s and dry 5. Proper isolation 6. Pretreat tooth surfaces 7. Light-cure or dual-cure composite resin luting agent
Polymer-infiltrated ceramic network	1. Intraoral restoration try-in 2. Etch with 9.8% HF acid for 1 min, rinse, and dry 3. Ultrasonic cleaning in alcohol for 5 min 4. Silane application for 20 s and dry 5. Proper isolation 6. Pretreat tooth surfaces 7. Light-cure or dual-cure composite resin luting agent
Y-TZP zirconia	1. Intraoral restoration try-in 2. Ultrasonic cleaning in alcohol for 5 min 3. APA with 50 μm alumina at 2 bar pressure 4. Application of special phosphate monomer-based primer 5. Proper isolation method 6. Pretreat tooth surfaces 7. Dual-cure or self-cure composite resin luting agent

their zirconia restorations. Cleaning agents, such as Ivoclean (Ivoclar Vivadent, Schaan, Liechtenstein), Katana Cleaner (Kuraray Noritake Dental), and ZirClean (BISCO Dental, Schaumburg, IL), are effective in removing contaminants and proteins from bonding surfaces of ceramics and other restorative materials after intraoral try-in.[131,132] Ivoclean is an alkaline suspension of zirconium oxide particles. Phosphate contaminants in saliva bond to those particles rather than to the restoration surface after suspension application and get washed off during the subsequent rinsing step. ZirClean is a potassium hydroxide–containing alkaline solution (pH 13), which similarly removes phosphate contaminants. In contrast, the cleaning effectiveness of Katana Cleaner is caused by surface active characteristics of its MDP salt. Besides application to various dental materials, this agent can also be used to clean tooth surfaces intraorally, because of its mild pH.

Table 1 summarizes recommended bonding protocols for dental ceramics.

SUMMARY

The longevity of resin-bonded ceramic restorations depends on the quality and durability of the resin-ceramic bonding interface. The type and composition of a specific ceramic material determines the selection of the most effective bonding protocol. Such protocol typically includes a surface pretreatment step followed by application of a priming agent to ensure strong and long-term durable resin bonds.

CLINICS CARE POINTS

- Silica-based ceramics should be acid etched with hydrofluoric (HF) acid based on their specific composition, followed by application of a silane coupling agent.
- Polymer-infiltrated ceramic network materials should ideally be HF acid etched and pretreated with a silane coupling agent.
- Metal-oxide ceramic such as zirconia require air-particle abrasion and application of a primer containing adhesive phosphate monomers for long-term durable bond strengths.
- Proper intraoral isolation of the working field is essential for resin-bonding procedures.

REFERENCES

1. Mizrahi B. The anterior all-ceramic crown: a rationale for the choice of ceramic and cement. Br Dent J 2008;205:251–5.
2. Rekow E, Silva N, Coelho P, et al. Performance of dental ceramics: challenges for improvements. J Dent Res 2011;90:937–52.
3. El-Mowafy O. The use of resin cements in restorative dentistry to overcome retention problems. J Can Dent Assoc 2001;67:97–102.
4. Sorensen J, Kang S, Avera S. Porcelain-composite interface microleakage with various porcelain surface treatments. Dent Mater 1991;7:118–23.
5. Blatz MB, Sadan A, Kern M. Resin-ceramic bonding: a review of the literature. J Prosthet Dent 2003;89:268–74.
6. Krämer N, Lohbauer U, Frankenberger R. Adhesive luting of indirect restorations. Am J Dent 2000;13:60D–76D.
7. Thompson JY, Stoner BR, Piascik JR, et al. Adhesion/cementation to zirconia and other non-silicate ceramics: where are we now? Dent Mater 2011;27:71–82.

8. Oyagüe RC, Monticelli F, Toledano M, et al. Effect of water aging on microtensile bond strength of dual-cured resin cements to pre-treated sintered zirconium-oxide ceramics. Dent Mater 2009;2:392–9.

9. Tian T, Tsoi JK-H, Matinlinna JP, et al. Aspects of bonding between resin luting cements and glass ceramic materials. Dent Mater 2014;30:e147–62.

10. Haddad MF, Rocha EP, Assunção WG. Cementation of prosthetic restorations: from conventional cementation to dental bonding concept. J Craniofac Surg 2011;22:952–8.

11. Rosenstiel SF, Land MF, Crispin BJ. Dental luting agents: a review of the current literature. J Prosthet Dent 1998;80:280–301.

12. Makkar S, Malhotra N. Self-adhesive resin cements: a new perspective in luting technology. Dent Update 2013;40:758–68.

13. Benetti AR, Papia E, Matinlinna JP. Bonding ceramic restorations. Nor Tannlege-foren Tid 2019;129:30–6.

14. Sideridou ID, Achilias DS. Elution study of unreacted Bis-GMA, TEGDMA, UDMA, and Bis-EMA from light-cured dental resins and resin composites using HPLC. J Biomed Mater Res 2005;74:617–26.

15. de Lima E, Santos R, Durão M, et al. Universal cements: dual activated and chemically activated. Acta Biomater Odontol Scand 2016;2:125–9.

16. Alammar A, Att W. Bonding durability between zirconia and different types of tooth or implant abutments-a systematic review. Part I: outcomes of in vitro studies. Int J Prosthodont 2021;34:650–69.

17. Klosa K, Meyer G, Kern M. Clinically used adhesive ceramic bonding methods: a survey in 2007, 2011, and in 2015. Clin Oral Investig 2016;20:1691–8.

18. Kern M. Bonding to oxide ceramics: laboratory testing versus clinical outcome. Dent Mater 2015;31:8–14.

19. Vargas MA, Bergeron C, Diaz-Arnold A. Cementing all-ceramic restorations: recommendations for success. J Am Dent Assoc 2011;142:20S–4S.

20. Subramanian D. All ceramic cementation protocols and resin cements for bonding: a key to success. JIDAM 2019;6:58–65.

21. Kelly JR, Nishimura I, Campbell SD. Ceramics in dentistry: historical roots and current perspectives. J Prosthet Dent 1996;75:18–32.

22. Mishra P, Mantri SS, Deogade S, et al. Richmond crown: a lost state of art. Int J Oral Health Sci 2015;2:448–53.

23. Helvey GA. Classification of dental ceramics. Inside Continuing Educ 2013; 13:62–8.

24. Anusavice KJ, Shen C, Rawls HR. Phillips' science of dental materials. Amsterdam, Netherlands: Elsevier Health Sciences; 2012.

25. Pollington S, van Noort R. An update of ceramics in dentistry. Int J Clin Dent 2009;2:283–307.

26. Conejo J, Nueesch R, Vonderheide M, et al. Clinical performance of all-ceramic dental restorations. Curr Oral Health Rep 2017;4:112–23.

27. Morimoto S, Rebello de Sampaio F, Braga M, et al. Survival rate of resin and ceramic inlays, onlays, and overlays: a systematic review and meta-analysis. J Dent Res 2016;95:985–94.

28. Frankenberger R, Taschner M, Garcia-Godoy F, et al. Leucite-reinforced glass ceramic inlays and onlays after 12 years. J Adhes Dent 2008;10:393–8.

29. Abduo J, Sambrook RJ. Longevity of ceramic onlays: a systematic review. J Esthet Dent 2018;30:193–215.

30. Yildiz C, Vanlıoğlu BA, Evren B, et al. Fracture resistance of manually and CAD/CAM manufactured ceramic onlays. J Prosthodont 2013;22:537–42.

31. Stappert CF, Ozden U, Gerds T, et al. Longevity and failure load of ceramic veneers with different preparation designs after exposure to masticatory simulation. J Prosthet Dent 2005;94:132–9.

32. da Cunha LF, Reis R, Santana L, et al. Ceramic veneers with minimum preparation. Eur J Dent 2013;7:492–6.

33. Kern M, Sasse M. Ten-year survival of anterior all-ceramic resin-bonded fixed dental prostheses. J Adhes Dent 2011;13:407.

34. Sasse M, Kern M. Survival of anterior cantilevered all-ceramic resin-bonded fixed dental prostheses made from zirconia ceramic. J Dent 2014;42:660–3.

35. Tabatabaian F, Taghizade F, Namdari M. Effect of coping thickness and background type on the masking ability of a zirconia ceramic. J Prosthet Dent 2018;119:159–65.

36. Ha S-J, Cho J-H. Comparison of the fit accuracy of zirconia-based prostheses generated by two CAD/CAM systems. J Adv Prosthodont 2016;8:439–48.

37. Contrepois M, Soenen A, Bartala M, et al. Marginal adaptation of ceramic crowns: a systematic review. J Prosthet Dent 2013;110:447–54.e10.

38. Tabata LF, de Lima Silva TA, de Paula Silveira AC, et al. Marginal and internal fit of CAD-CAM composite resin and ceramic crowns before and after internal adjustment. J Prosthet Dent 2020;123:500–5.

39. Tinschert J, Natt G, Mautsch W, et al. Marginal fit of alumina-and zirconia-based fixed partial dentures produced by a CAD/CAM system. Oper 2001;26:367–74.

40. Pilathadka S, Vahalová D, Vosáhlo T. The zirconia: a new dental ceramic material. An overview. Prague Med Rep 2007;108:5–12.

41. Chrcanovic BR, Kisch J, Larsson C. Retrospective clinical evaluation of 2- to 6-unit implant-supported fixed partial dentures: mean follow-up of 9 years. Clin Implant Dent Relat Res 2020;22:201–12.

42. Nazari V, Ghodsi S, Alikhasi M, et al. Fracture strength of three-unit implant supported fixed partial dentures with excessive crown height fabricated from different materials. J Dent 2016;13:400.

43. Blatz M, Vonderheide M, Conejo J. The effect of resin bonding on long-term success of high-strength ceramics. J Dent Res 2018;97:132–9.

44. Kern M. Resin bonding to oxide ceramics for dental restorations. J Adhes Sci Technol 2009;23:1097–111.

45. Blatz MB, Conejo J. The current state of chairside digital dentistry and materials. Dent Clin N AM 2019;63:175–97.

46. Höland W, Rheinberger V, Apel E, et al. Future perspectives of biomaterials for dental restoration. J Eur Ceram Soc 2009;29:1291–7.

47. Beier US, Dumfahrt H. Longevity of silicate ceramic restorations. Quintessence Int 2014;45:701–9.

48. Powers JM, Farah JW, O'Keefe KL, et al. Guide to all-ceramic bonding. Dent Advis 2009;2:1–12.

49. Sailer I, Makarov NA, Thoma DS, et al. All-ceramic or metal-ceramic tooth-supported fixed dental prostheses (FDPs)? A systematic review of the survival and complication rates. Part I: single crowns (SCs). Dent Mater 2015;31:603–23.

50. Alenezi A, Alsweed M, Alsidrani S, et al. Long-term survival and complication rates of porcelain laminate veneers in clinical studies: a systematic review. J Clin Med 2021;10:1074.

51. Otto T, Schneider D. Long-term clinical results of chairside Cerec CAD/CAM inlays and onlays: a case series. Int J Prosthodont 2008;21:53–9.

52. Del Rio DL, Sandoval-Sanchez E, Campos-Villegas NE, et al. Influence of heated hydrofluoric acid surface treatment on surface roughness and bond strength

to feldspathic ceramics and lithium-disilicate glass-ceramics. J Adhes Dent 2021;23:549–55.

53. Prochnow C, Pereira GKR, Venturini AB, et al. How does hydrofluoric acid etching affect the cyclic load-to-failure of lithium disilicate restorations? J Mech Behav Biomed Mater 2018;87:306–11.

54. Prochnow C, Venturini AB, Grasel R, et al. Adhesion to a lithium disilicate glass ceramic etched with hydrofluoric acid at distinct concentrations. Braz Dent J 2018;29:492–9.

55. Barjaktarova-Valjakova E, Grozdanov A, Guguvcevski L, et al. Acid etching as surface treatment method for luting of glass-ceramic restorations, part 1: acids, application protocol and etching effectiveness. Open Acess Maced 2018;6:568–73.

56. Venturini AB, Prochnow C, Rambo D, et al. Effect of hydrofluoric acid concentration on resin adhesion to a feldspathic ceramic. J Adhes Dent 2015;17:313–20.

57. Sundfeld D, Palialol ARM, Fugolin APP, et al. The effect of hydrofluoric acid and resin cement formulation on the bond strength to lithium disilicate ceramic. Braz Oral Res 2018;32:e43.

58. Mangani F, Cerutti A, Putignano A, et al. Clinical approach to anterior adhesive restorations using resin composite veneers. Eur J Esthet Dent 2007;2:188–209.

59. Novais VR, Raposo LHA, Miranda RRD, et al. Degree of conversion and bond strength of resin-cements to feldspathic ceramic using different curing modes. J Appl Oral Sci 2017;25:61–8.

60. Kowalska A, Sokolowski J, Bociong K. The photoinitiators used in resin based dental composite: a review and future perspectives. Polym J 2021;13:470.

61. Tripodakis AP, Kaitsas V, Putignano A, et al. Proceedings of the 2011 Autumn meeting of the EAED (active members' meeting)-Versailles, October 20-22nd, 2011. Eur J Dent 2012;7:186–241.

62. Faria-e-Silva AL, Pfeifer CS. Development of dual-cured resin cements with long working time, high conversion in absence of light and reduced polymerization stress. Dent Mater 2020;36:e293–301.

63. Yang Y, Wang Y, Yang H, et al. Effect of aging on color stability and bond strength of dual-cured resin cement with amine or amine-free self-initiators. Dent Mater 2022;41(1):17–26.

64. Prieto LT, de Araújo CTP, Pierote JJA, et al. Evaluation of degree of conversion and the effect of thermal aging on the color stability of resin cements and flowable composite. J Conserv Dent 2018;21:47–51.

65. Tagami A, Takahashi R, Nikaido T, et al. The effect of curing conditions on the dentin bond strength of two dual-cure resin cements. J Prosthodont Res 2017;61:412–8.

66. Farias DCS, Gonçalves LM, Walter R, et al. Bond strengths of various resin cements to different ceramics. Braz Oral Res 2019;33:e95.

67. Khudair H, Alnajjar B. Effect of bonding technique on microleakage around ceramic laminate veneers (in-vitro comparative study). Int J Appl Dent Sci 2020;6:247–53.

68. Cattell M, Chadwick T, Knowles J, et al. Flexural strength optimisation of a leucite reinforced glass ceramic. Dent Mater 2001;17:21–33.

69. Nejatidanesh F, Amjadi M, Akouchekian M, et al. Clinical performance of CEREC AC Bluecam conservative ceramic restorations after five years: a retrospective study. J Dent 2015;43:1076–82.

70. Fradeani M, Redemagni M. An 11-year clinical evaluation of leucite-reinforced glass-ceramic crowns: a retrospective study. Quintessence Int 2002;33:503–10.

71. do Amaral Colombo L, Murillo-Gomez F, De Goes MF. Bond strength of CAD/CAM restorative materials treated with different surface etching protocols. J Adhes Dent 2019;21:307–17.

72. Straface A, Rupp L, Gintaute A, et al. HF etching of CAD/CAM materials: influence of HF concentration and etching time on shear bond strength. Head Face Med 2019;15:1–10.

73. Veríssimo AH, Moura DMD, Tribst JPM, et al. Effect of hydrofluoric acid concentration and etching time on resin-bond strength to different glass ceramics. Braz Oral Res 2019;33:e41.

74. Gracis S, Thompson VP, Ferencz JL, et al. A new classification system for all-ceramic and ceramic-like restorative materials. Int J Prosthodont 2015;28: 227–35.

75. Malament KA, Margvelashvili-Malament M, Natto ZS, et al. Comparison of 16.9-year survival of pressed acid etched e.max lithium disilicate glass ceramic complete and partial coverage restorations in posterior teeth: performance and outcomes as a function of tooth position, age, sex, and thickness of ceramic material. J Prosthet Dent 2020;126:533–45.

76. Reich S, Schierz O. Chair-side generated posterior lithium disilicate crowns after 4 years. Clin Oral Investig 2013;17:1765–72.

77. Van Den Breemer C, Gresnigt M, Özcan M, et al. Prospective randomized clinical trial on the survival of lithium disilicate posterior partial crowns bonded using immediate or delayed dentin sealing: short-term results on tooth sensitivity and patient satisfaction. Oper 2019;44:e212–22.

78. Vichi A, Fabian Fonzar R, Carrabba M, et al. Comparison between hydrofluoric acid and single-component primer as conditioners on resin cement adhesion to lithium silicate and lithium disilicate glass ceramics. Mater 2021;14:6776.

79. Li R, Ma SQ, Zang CC, et al. Enhanced bonding strength between lithium disilicate ceramics and resin cement by multiple surface treatments after thermal cycling. PLoS One 2019;14:e0220466.

80. Fasbinder DJ, Dennison JB, Heys D, et al. A clinical evaluation of chairside lithium disilicate CAD/CAM crowns. J Am Dent Assoc 2010;141:10S–4S.

81. Rigolin FJ, Miranda ME, Florio FM, et al. Evaluation of bond strength between leucite-based and lithium disilicate-based ceramics to dentin after cementation with conventional and self-adhesive resin agents. Acta Odontol Latinoam 2014; 27:16–24.

82. Cardenas AM, Siqueira F, Hass V, et al. Effect of MDP-containing silane and adhesive used alone or in combination on the long-term bond strength and chemical interaction with lithium disilicate ceramics. J Adhes Dent 2017;19:203–12.

83. Nagarkar S, Theis-Mahon N, Perdigão J. Universal dental adhesives: current status, laboratory testing, and clinical performance. J Biomed Mater Res B Appl Biomater 2019;107:2121–31.

84. Özcan M, Volpato CÂM. Surface conditioning and bonding protocol for polymer-infiltrated ceramic: how and why? J Adhes Dent 2016;18:174–5.

85. Swain M, Coldea A, Bilkhair A, et al. Interpenetrating network ceramic-resin composite dental restorative materials. Dent Mater 2016;32:34–42.

86. He L-H, Swain M. A novel polymer infiltrated ceramic dental material. Dent Mater 2011;27:527–34.

87. Conejo J, Ozer F, Mante F, et al. Effect of surface treatment and cleaning on the bond strength to polymer-infiltrated ceramic network CAD-CAM material. J Prosthet Dent 2021;126:698–702.

88. Bottino M, Campos F, Ramos N, et al. Inlays made from a hybrid material: adaptation and bond strengths. Oper 2015;40:E83–91.
89. Mörmann WH, Stawarczyk B, Ender A, et al. Wear characteristics of current aesthetic dental restorative CAD/CAM materials: two-body wear, gloss retention, roughness and Martens hardness. J Mech Behav Biomed Mater 2013;20: 113–25.
90. Della Bona A, Corazza PH, Zhang Y. Characterization of a polymer-infiltrated ceramic-network material. Dent Mater 2014;30:564–9.
91. Emsermann I, Eggmann F, Krastl G, et al. Influence of pretreatment methods on the adhesion of composite and polymer infiltrated ceramic CAD-CAM blocks. J Adhes Dent 2019;21:433–43.
92. Bello YD, Di Domenico MB, Magro LD, et al. Bond strength between composite repair and polymer-infiltrated ceramic-network material: effect of different surface treatments. J Esthet Dent 2019;31:275–9.
93. Spitznagel FA, Horvath SD, Guess PC, et al. Resin bond to indirect composite and new ceramic/polymer materials: a review of the literature. J Esthet Dent 2014;26:382–93.
94. Hu M, Weiger R, Fischer J. Comparison of two test designs for evaluating the shear bond strength of resin composite cements. Dent Mater 2016;32:223–32.
95. Elsaka SE. Repair bond strength of resin composite to a novel CAD/CAM hybrid ceramic using different repair systems. Dent Mater J 2015;34:161–7.
96. Mühlemann S, Lakha T, Jung RE, et al. Prosthetic outcomes and clinical performance of CAD-CAM monolithic zirconia versus porcelain-fused-to-metal implant crowns in the molar region: 1-year results of a RCT. Clin Oral Implants Res 2020; 31:856–64.
97. Spitznagel F, Boldt J, Gierthmuehlen P. CAD/CAM ceramic restorative materials for natural teeth. J Dent Res 2018;97:1082–91.
98. Lawson NC, Maharishi A. Strength and translucency of zirconia after high-speed sintering. J Esthet Dent 2020;32:219–25.
99. Jansen JU, Lümkemann N, Letz I, et al. Impact of high-speed sintering on translucency, phase content, grain sizes, and flexural strength of 3Y-TZP and 4Y-TZP zirconia materials. J Prosthet Dent 2019;122:396–403.
100. Lümkemann N, Pfefferle R, Jerman E, et al. Translucency, flexural strength, fracture toughness, fracture load of 3-unit FDPs, martens hardness parameter and grain size of 3Y-TZP materials. Dent Mater 2020;36:838–45.
101. Zhang F, Van Meerbeek B, Vleugels J. Importance of tetragonal phase in high-translucent partially stabilized zirconia for dental restorations. Dent Mater 2020; 36:491–500.
102. Jerman E, Lümkemann N, Eichberger M, et al. Evaluation of translucency, Marten's hardness, biaxial flexural strength and fracture toughness of 3Y-TZP, 4Y-TZP and 5Y-TZP materials. Dent Mater 2021;37:212–22.
103. Inokoshi M, Shimizu H, Nozaki K, et al. Crystallographic and morphological analysis of sandblasted highly translucent dental zirconia. Dent Mater 2018; 34:508–18.
104. Kelly JR Denry I. Stabilized zirconia as a structural ceramic: an overview. Dent Mater 2008;24:289–98.
105. Scaminaci Russo D, Cinelli F, Sarti C, et al. Adhesion to zirconia: a systematic review of current conditioning methods and bonding materials. J Dent 2019; 7:74.
106. Quigley NP, Loo DS, Choy C, et al. Clinical efficacy of methods for bonding to zirconia: a systematic review. J Prosthet Dent 2021;125:231–40.

107. Levartovsky S, Cartier L, Brand M, et al. The retentive strength of zirconium oxide crowns cemented by self-adhesive resin cements before and after 6 months of aging. Mater 2020;13:3998.

108. Comino-Garayoa R, Peláez J, Tobar C, et al. Adhesion to zirconia: a systematic review of surface pretreatments and resin cements. Mater 2021;14:2751.

109. Elraggal A, Silikas N. Effect of air-abraded versus laser-fused fluorapatite glass-ceramics on shear bond strength of repair materials to zirconia. Mater 2021;14:1468.

110. Hamdy AM, Hashem ABH. Effect of surface treatment and artificial aging on microtensile bond strength of zirconia to resin cement. Egypt Dent J 2017;63:2487–94.

111. Blatz MB, Alvarez M, Sawyer K, et al. How to bond zirconia: the APC concept. Compend Contin Educ Dent 2016;37:611–8.

112. Alammar A, Att W. Bonding durability between zirconia and different types of tooth or implant abutments-a systematic review. Part II: outcomes of in vitro studies. Int J Prosthodont 2021;34(5):650–69.

113. Güth J-F, Stawarczyk B, Edelhoff D, et al. Zirconia and its novel compositions: what do clinicians need to know? Quintessence Int 2019;50:512–20.

114. Spies BC, Zhang F, Wesemann C, et al. Reliability and aging behavior of three different zirconia grades used for monolithic four-unit fixed dental prostheses. Dent Mater 2020;36:e329–39.

115. Holman CD, Lien W, Gallardo FF, et al. Assessing flexural strength degradation of new cubic containing zirconia materials. J Contemp Dent 2020;21:114–8.

116. Rabel K, Lamott U, Polydorou O, et al. Prosthodontic rehabilitation with fixed monolithic translucent zirconia restorations: a case history report. Int J Prosthodont 2019;32:544–8.

117. Souza R, Barbosa F, Araújo G, et al. Ultrathin monolithic zirconia veneers: reality or future? Report of a clinical case and one-year follow-up. Oper 2018;43:3–11.

118. McLaren EA, Lawson N, Choi J, et al. New high-translucent cubic-phase–containing zirconia: clinical and laboratory considerations and the effect of air abrasion on strength. Compend 2017;38:e13–7.

119. Franco-Tabares S, Wardecki D, Nakamura K, et al. Effect of airborne-particle abrasion and polishing on novel translucent zirconias: surface morphology, phase transformation and insights into bonding. J Prosthodont Res 2021;65:97–105.

120. Mehari K, Parke AS, Gallardo FF, et al. Assessing the effects of air abrasion with aluminum oxide or glass beads to zirconia on the bond strength of cement. J Contemp Dent 2020;21:713–7.

121. Franco-Tabares S, Stenport VF, Hjalmarsson L, et al. Chemical bonding to novel translucent zirconias: a mechanical and molecular investigation. J Adhes Dent 2019;21:107–16.

122. Ruales-Carrera E, Cesar PF, Henriques B, et al. Adhesion behavior of conventional and high-translucent zirconia: effect of surface conditioning methods and aging using an experimental methodology. J Esthet Dent 2019;31:388–97.

123. Chen B, Yan Y, Xie H, et al. Effects of tribochemical silica coating and alumina-particle air abrasion on 3Y-TZP and 5Y-TZP: evaluation of surface hardness, roughness, bonding, and phase transformation. J Adhes Dent 2020;22:373–82.

124. Shimizu H, Inokoshi M, Takagaki T, et al. Bonding efficacy of 4-META/MMA-TBB resin to surface-treated highly translucent dental zirconia. J Adhes Dent 2018;20:453–9.

125. Sakrana A, Al-Zordk W, Shoukry H, et al. Bond strength durability of adhesive cements to translucent zirconia: effect of surface conditioning. Eur J Prosthodont Restor Dent 2020;28:161–71.
126. Alammar A, Blatz MB. The resin bond to high-translucent zirconia: a systematic review. J Esthet Dent 2022;34(1):117–35.
127. Khanlar LN, Takagaki T, Abdou A, et al. Effect of Air-Particle Abrasion Protocol and Primer on The Topography and Bond Strength of a High-Translucent Zirconia Ceramic. J Prosthodont 2021;31(3):228–38.
128. Schuh PL, Wachtel H, Bolz W, et al. Teflon tape technique": synergy between isolation and lucidity. Quintessence Int 2019;50:488–93.
129. Browet S, Gerdolle D. Precision and security in restorative dentistry: the synergy of isolation and magnification. Int J Esthet Dent 2017;12:172–85.
130. Al-Akhali M, Al-Dobaei E, Wille S, et al. Influence of elapsed time between airborne-particle abrasion and bonding to zirconia bond strength. Dent Mater 2021;37:516–22.
131. Wattanasirmkit K, Charasseangpaisarn T. Effect of different cleansing agents and adhesive resins on bond strength of contaminated zirconia. J Prosthodont Res 2019;63:271–6.
132. Alex G. Zirconia: separating fact from fiction. Oral Health 2019;9(7):60–1.

Dental Implants

Enhancing Biological Response Through Surface Modifications

In-Sung Luke Yeo, DDS, MS, PhD

KEYWORDS

- Dental implants • Bone-implant interface • Osseointegration • Micro-topography
- Nano-topography • Wettability • Chemical modification • Biofunctionalization

KEY POINTS

- Topographic, physical, or chemical modification of a dental implant surface enhances biological response, particularly bone-healing response to the modified surface.
- The micro-topographical modification of an implant surface enhances bone response, which occurs by mimicking the resorption pits by osteoclasts on natural bone surfaces. Two representative modified surfaces of grade 4 commercially pure titanium, sandblasted, large-grit, acid-etched, and electrochemically oxidized surfaces have been evidenced in the clinical long-term implant survival.
- Nano-modifications of implant surfaces include alterations of the topographic, chemical, and physical properties. These nano-alterations are usually combined with micromodifications and warrant further clinical investigation.
- The application of biofunctional molecules to implant surfaces seems promising because of their potential to alter the bone-healing capacity of the local environment surrounding the implant, which would be beneficial to patients with compromised bone metabolism who are contraindicated for an implant treatment.

INTRODUCTION

The characteristics of implant surfaces are key factors for long-term clinical success.[1] Since the 1970s, dental implant surfaces have changed in clinical application from the machine-turned surface of grade 1 commercially pure titanium (cp-Ti) to the micro-roughened surface of grade 4 cp-Ti or grade 5 Ti alloy.[2,3] Nanostructural modifications (arithmetical mean roughness over the surface, or Sa, between 1 and 100 nm), chemical modifications, or wettability control technology are applied to dental implant surfaces based on roughening methods at the microlevel (Sa between 1 and 10 μm).[2–5] Recently, the aforementioned techniques have modified the surfaces of new

Department of Prosthodontics, School of Dentistry and Dental Research Institute, Seoul National University, 101 Daehak-Ro, Jongro-Gu, Seoul 03080, Korea
E-mail address: pros53@snu.ac.kr

Dent Clin N Am 66 (2022) 627–642
https://doi.org/10.1016/j.cden.2022.05.009
0011-8532/22/© 2022 The Author. Published by Elsevier Inc.

biomedical materials, including zirconia and tantalum, for their use as an oral implant, despite cp-Ti or Ti alloy being the materials of choice.[6–11]

Although a screw-shaped dental implant is prepared by milling with a computer numerical control machine, its original surface is a basic surface without modifications.[3] It is called a turned surface, and the turned cp-Ti surfaces had been actively used in clinical implant dentistry until the 1990s.[12–15] The introduction of surface modifications to an endosseous screw-shaped dental implant began with changes in surface topography and roughness, along with the application of both physical and chemical modifications by hydroxyapatite to cylinder-shaped implants.[16,17] The sandblasted, large-grit, acid-etched (SLA) Ti surface and the anodically oxidized Ti surface are two major surface modifications that are topographically different at the microlevel and widely used clinically. Since the 1990s, nano-approaches to the modification of dental implant surfaces have been investigated.[5,18–22] Initially, the effect of nano-modification was questionable because complete bone ingrowth does not occur in spaces considerably smaller than 100 μm.[23] Considering the dimensions of an osteon and the response of bone ground substances to surface micro-irregularities, it is difficult to show evidence for nano-modifications in enhancing the bone response.[24,25] However, surface nano-topography and chemistry have been reported to affect protein adsorption, osteogenic cell behavior, and bone–implant interaction.[2,26–31]

Proposing modifications of dental implant surfaces require an understanding of the nature of osseointegration. Osseointegration was originally a phenomenological term, defined as the direct contact between a bone and the implant surface, visualized through light microscopy.[1] Considering this definition, the biocompatibility of a material in contact with the bone was a major issue while investigating the formation of bone surrounding implants.[3,22] Surface modification at the level of micro-topography and micro-roughness focused on quantitating bone apposition. However, the modifications also altered cellular behavior in vitro and bone physiology in vivo.[4,32,33] Osseointegration is considered a type of bone healing with an inflammatory response,[22,34] and a dental implant surface has been modified in its nano-topography, surface chemistry, and surface energy to enhance the healing.[2,27,29,35–37]

A dental implant system inserted into a patient's mouth comprises five interfaces associated with a biological response. The suprastructure interface to the oral cavity and the suprastructure–abutment interface in the salivary environment are both considered to be present outside the body, which involves numerous factors. The soft tissue–abutment interface is in the transgingival region, a special area connecting the outside and inside of the body. The biological response to this interface necessitates understanding another interface, an implant–abutment interface.[15,38] The last is the bone–implant interface in the body. This review briefly explores surface modifications of dental implants designed to enhance hard tissue response at the bone–implant interface. This article deals with healing physiology around implants and interactions between the bone and the characteristics of modified implant surfaces.

HEALING PROCESS SURROUNDING DENTAL IMPLANTS

Drilling a hole for implant insertion in dental surgery leads to bleeding and hemostasis in the bone from surgical trauma, which lasts for minutes to hours. The procedure of implant drilling generates bone debris which releases various cytokines and bone matrix proteins activated by the trauma.[39] Bleeding and damaged endothelium from injured blood vessels form platelet plugs, simultaneously provoking the coagulation cascade toward hemostasis.[40,41] The surface of an implant initially contacts blood during the implant insertion into the hole. Surface wettability, charge, and topography play an important role in initial bone healing.[5,29,32,42] Protein adsorption occurs on the surface; initially, this is by high mobility proteins at higher concentration in the plasma, which are then replaced by other proteins having a higher affinity for the implant surface (Vroman effect) (**Fig. 1**A).[40,43] This process gets delayed on a hydrophobic surface, thus highlighting the importance of a hydrophilic surface in preserving the tertiary structures and activities of proteins adsorbed on the surface.[40,43] Mesenchymal stem cells subsequently bind to the adsorbed extracellular matrix proteins (ECMs), which include fibronectin and vitronectin.[4,40,42]

Vitronectin on the implant surface binds platelets and activates them, thus forming a platelet plug.[40] This plug binds thrombocytes, resulting in their degranulation. Such platelet degranulation releases growth factors and causes cytokine degranulation, thus leading to the inflammatory phase that begins after approximately 10 minutes and lasts for some days following the implant installation surgery.[40] Neutrophils indicate acute inflammation, and the presence of mononuclear cells implies that wound healing around the dental implant is in the chronic inflammatory stage (**Fig. 1**B).[44] These inflammatory responses usually subside at a biocompatible interface within 2 weeks.[44] Subsequently, macrophages arrive at the implant site and adhere to the dental implant surface, with some fusing to form foreign-body giant cells. The aforementioned adhesion and fusion are supported by vitronectin via integrins, the transmembrane proteins of cells, which implies that granulation tissue is forming at the bone–implant interface.[44–47]

Granulation tissue is identified by new extracellular matrix, fibroblast infiltration, and neovascularization.[40,44] Macrophages are activated by certain physical and chemical properties of implant surfaces.[48] These macrophages stimulate fibrogenesis by fibroblasts, an essential component in wound healing (**Fig. 1**C).[41,44,49] Various cytokines released from the macrophages contribute to wound healing, as does the primary

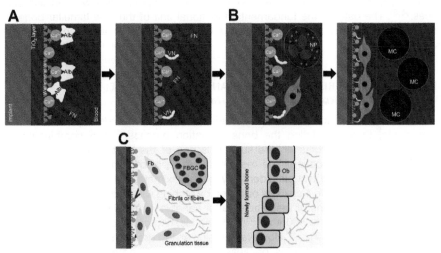

Fig. 1. Bone healing on an implant surface. (*A*) Initial adhesion on the surface is by plasma proteins in higher concentration, such as albumin. Later, higher affinitive proteins (fibronectin, vitronectin, and so forth) replace them. (*B*) Inflammatory phase. Neutrophils and mononuclear cells are found in this stage. (*C*) Stimulation by foreign-body giant cells, fibrogenesis, and various cytokines differentiate mesenchymal stem cells into osteoblasts that form new bone around the implant surface. Alb, albumin; Fb, fibroblast; FBGC, foreign-body giant cell; FN, fibronectin; MC, mononuclear cell; MsC, mesenchymal stem cell; NP, neutrophil; Ob, osteoblast; VN, vitronectin.

stability of the implants.[40,44] The loss of primary stability, or micromovement, of the implant produces shear stress that disrupts normal bone healing.[40] Simultaneous angiogenesis occurs at the wound site, which is stimulated by macrophage-secreted molecules.[40,44] Bone morphogenetic proteins (BMPs) are stored in and released from the old bone matrix and drive new bone formation.[40,50] They are activated by bone trauma, such as implant drilling, and stimulate the differentiation of mesenchymal stem cells into osteoblasts.[40] Newly formed bone, also known as woven bone, then establishes contact with the implant surface, typically 1-week post-implant placement when the surface has been modified (see **Fig. 1C**).[32,51]

Bone remodeling matures the woven bone into lamellar or compact bone. This process can continue for years depending on the load distribution around the implant and the strain induced within the bone.[40,52] This load distribution and bone strain are more affected by the implant geometry and the implant–abutment connection structure than by the implant surface quality.[15,38] Osteoclasts play an important role in bone remodeling by providing space for the lamellar bone. Bone resorption by osteoclasts is balanced with bone formation by osteoblasts.[40,41] The osteogenic cells lining the cement line dissolve the osteoid with collagenases, thereby exposing RGD (tripeptide arginine, glycine, and aspartate) endings from the surface and causing cell detachment.[40,53] Migrating osteoclast precursors are attracted by the recently exposed bone surface and become attached. These precursors differentiate into osteoclasts, which are phenotypically different multinucleated giant cells, and form a resorption apparatus, also termed ruffled borders. This in turn seals the margin and the Howship's lacuna where the mineralized bone matrix gets disintegrated.[40,44,54] Osteogenic cells are able to recognize the texture of the bone surface in the lacuna.[55,56] These cells obtain information about the bone quantity necessary to fill the lacuna.[56] The aforementioned characteristic may be involved in the enhanced osteogenic activity of the cells by sensing the irregularities of micro-topographically modified surfaces.[55,57] The osteon, the fundamental functional unit of the new lamellar bone, is formed to effectively withstand the load transferred via the endosseous screw-shaped implant.

IMPLANT SURFACE TREATMENTS TO ENHANCE BONE RESPONSE
Modifications for Micro-topographical Surface Change

Methods to micro-roughen the implant surface mimic the resorption pits created by osteoclasts, thus stimulating the bone formation process.[55] The combination of acid-etching and sandblasting the surface is one of the best known methods for implant surface modification. The resulting surface, also termed the SLA surface, has been clinically used in implant dentistry for approximately 30 years.[58–60] Generally, an SLA surface on grade 4 cp- Ti is obtained by etching with hydrochloric, sulfuric, nitric acid or combinations of these acids after sandblasting the surface with alumina particles measuring 75 to 500 μm.[3,55,61,62] The blasting procedure on a zirconia surface is similar to that on Ti.[55,63] However, etching on the zirconia surface is usually performed with bases and not acids, because the polycrystalline zirconia is unaffected by acids, such as hydrogen fluoride (HF), which are typically used for dental ceramics containing a glassy matrix, such as porcelain.[55,63,64] The roughness (Sa) of commercial SLA surfaces is approximately 1.5 μm, which is considered optimal for bone healing.[25,29,47,65]

Anodic oxidation is another well-known method for the modification of a dental implant surface.[62] Because the anode is defined as the site of oxidation in an electrochemical cell, the term electrochemical oxidation is a more suitable description than anodic oxidation. When a Ti dental implant is configured as the anode in an electro-chemical cell, an applied electrical potential accelerates the oxidation of the implant surface such that the Ti oxide (TiO_2) layer on the surface thickens and becomes micro-roughened compared with the TiO_2 film spontaneously formed in the atmo-sphere.[3] This oxidized Ti surface has a microporous structure with multiple volcano-like irregularities.[41,66]

Micro-topographical features influence bone responses to implant surfaces because osteogenic cells recognize the topographic characteristics on the implant surface similar to the way they recognize sites of resorbed bone.[55,67] However, the ef-ficacy in bone healing of honeycomb- or crater-like microstructures resulting from SLA as compared with the volcano-like microporous irregularities resulting from oxidation is unknown (**Fig. 2**). Several studies involving in vivo comparisons of micro-topographically varied surfaces have not demonstrated significant histomorphometric differences, despite better efficacy of osteogenesis shown with implant surfaces that are morphologically similar to osteoclast resorption pits.[68–71] Furthermore, it is difficult to directly compare the surfaces clinically due to different implant design factors, including implant–abutment connection structures and implant thread shapes.[15,65]

Both types of micro-roughened Ti implant surfaces have displayed high long-term survival rates in clinical studies. Previous 10-year clinical studies reported that the sur-vival rates of SLA dental implants were greater than 95%.[72–74] For the oxidized sur-face, clinical investigations analyzed data obtained from clinical use for ≥ 10 years and also reported high survival rates.[13,75,76] Various other factors, including clinicians' skills and placement arch (maxilla or mandible), exert effects on the clinical success or survival of dental implants.[12,14] However, these two types of micro-roughened sur-faces have been shown to have greater reliability for long-term clinical use than the un-modified surface, when the modified surfaces are on grade 4 cp- Ti and roughness is within the optimum range (1–2 μm in S_a).[3,5,13,72,73,76,77]

Modifications for Nano-Topographical Surface Change

The effect of nano-modification of the implant surface is often questioned, because complete bone ingrowth does not occur in spaces considerably smaller than 100 μm.[23] Therefore, it is difficult to attribute accelerated osteogenesis to nano-modification, considering the dimensions of an osteon and the response of bone ground substance to surface micro-irregularities, which are 10 to 500 μm and 200

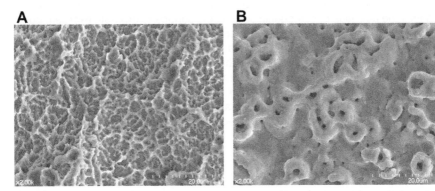

A   **B**

Fig. 2. Representative scanning electron microscopy (SEM) images of SLA (A) and oxidized (B) surfaces. The honeycomb-like appearance of the SLA and the volcano-like appearance of the oxidized surface are very different.

to 1000 μm for cortical and cancellous bones, respectively.[2,24,25] Nano-topography does not exert a notable effect on the responses of osteogenic cells or on the bone at the interfacial area.[78,79] However, surface nano-topography has recently demonstrated its usefulness in protein adsorption, osteogenic cell behavior, bone–implant interaction, drug delivery capability, and antibacterial action.[2,26–31,80,81] The nanotopographical characteristics of Ti implant surfaces affect the initial bone responses, including the activities of both osteoblasts and osteoclasts.[82,83]

By controlling the electric current, temperature, electrolyte concentration, oxidation voltage, and oxidation time in a fluoride-based solution, electrochemical oxidation can be used to nano-topographically produce a TiO_2 nanotube layer on the implant surface.[82,84] The TiO_2 nanotube-arrayed implant surface is highly biocompatible, despite the optimal nanotube diameter remaining under investigation.[82,85–88] Therefore, the modified surface has great potential in biologic and clinical applications. However, the TiO_2 nanotube-based surface has yet to be applied in the clinical situation. The interfacial bond strength between the TiO_2 nanotube layer and the underlying Ti surface is weak when exposed to frictional forces, such that the nanotube layer becomes easily delaminated on insertion of a nanotube-layered dental implant into the bone.[84]

Hydrophilicity

Water molecules establish the first contact with the implant surface during implant placement. Therefore, a hydrophilic surface is considered desirable for promoting the initial stages of bone healing.[3,5] The water-friendly surface of some successful dental implants comprises a hydrophilic SLA surface, termed modified SLA, or SLActive (Institute Straumann AG, Basel, Switzerland).[3] The SLActive surface maintains biological availability by retaining surface hydrophilicity, which is achieved by the prevention of hydrocarbon contamination during implant production and packaging.[5] This type of surface having a combination of wettability and micro-roughness has shown excellent long-term clinical success.[89]

Another approach to producing a hydrophilic implant surface is the decontamination of the surface by removal of the hydrocarbons that cause reduced biocompatibility.[90] Ultraviolet (UV) irradiation of implant surfaces to eliminate hydrocarbon contamination and increase surface hydrophilicity is particularly close to routine clinical use.[91] The wavelength of UV-C ranges from 200 to 280 nm and is most effective in the removal of carbon and contributing to excellent interfacial bone-healing results.[3,29] Without a notable nano-topographical change of an implant surface (**Fig. 3**), UV treatment increases the surface charge, improves the adsorption of plasma proteins, and enhances the activities of osteogenic cells on the surface to promote excellent bone-to-implant contact during in vivo experiments.[3,29,92] Despite few prospective clinical studies with observation periods ≥ 10 years, some prospective and retrospective clinical investigations have reported greater than 95% success rates of the UV-treated dental implant surfaces.[91,93] UV-treated turned Ti surfaces have demonstrated excellent bone-to-implant contact ratios, similar to those of micro-roughened SLA Ti surfaces, which are globally accepted in dental clinics. This type of photofunctionalized surface might be clinically more advantageous for the removal of biofilms on implant surfaces and in the treatment of peri-implantitis, compared with micro-roughened SLA and oxidized implant surfaces.[15,29,92]

Elemental Modifications on Surface

The application of chemicals with known osteogenic activity to an implant surface is another approach to nano-modification through surface chemistry. The coating of the implant surface by a calcium–phosphorus compound and the treatment of the

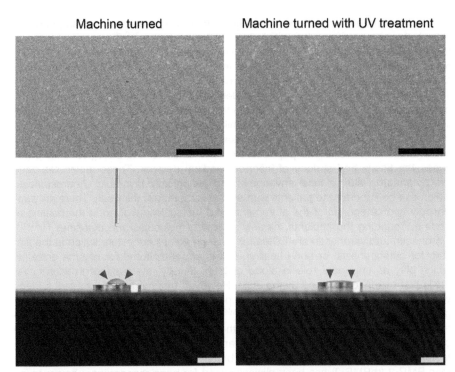

Fig. 3. In the SEM images of Ti discs (*top row*), little topographic difference is found after UV treatment. However, the contact angles (*bottom row*) indicating surface hydrophilicity are notably different (*blue arrowheads*). Scale bars = 500 μm.

surface with fluoride ion traces have been clinically applied to dental implants. In contrast, biologic molecules, such as proteins and functional peptides, have not yet been applied to implant surfaces and tested clinically.[3,27,28,47]

It is difficult to detect fluorides using energy dispersive spectroscopy. Small amounts of fluoride exist on a Ti implant surface reduced at the cathode in a low concentration of hydrofluoric acid solution in an electrochemical cell.[3] The fluoride ions are useful in bone mineralization and accelerate bone healing principally by stimulating undifferentiated osteogenic cells.[94] Micro-roughened Ti implant surfaces modified with a trace amount of fluoride have an average mean height or S_a within the optimal range of approximately 1.5 μm.[65] This fluoride-modified implant demonstrates high survival rates for long-term clinical service.[95] However, only one implant design has thus far been clinically used with this fluoride modification, and it is not yet known if the implant design itself or the surface characteristics are the key to clinical success.[15,96]

Calcium–phosphorus compounds, particularly hydroxyapatite, which is the principal component of human bone, are the major coating materials that have been tried for dental implants. Hydroxyapatite and other calcium–phosphorus materials are considered bioactive and osteoconductive to the surrounding bone.[3] However, the biodegradation of calcium–phosphorus particles caused by wear of the coating and the weak binding between the coating layer and underlying surface are major issues in the application of these coatings.[97] Researchers are developing various methods, including conventional plasma spraying, magnetron sputtering, and laser patterning to prepare more stable and biocompatible coating layers by controlling their physical topography, crystallinity, and calcium–phosphorus ratios (**Fig. 4**).[97–99] Previous animal studies have suggested that the hydroxyapatite coating accelerates osteogenesis at the interfacial area during the initial stage of bone healing.[100] The survival rates of hydroxyapatite-coated dental implants have been shown to be greater than 90% for 5 years or more, despite reports on rates less than 90%.[101,102] There are no clinical studies estimating the application of other calcium–phosphorus compounds to dental implant surfaces for long-term use. Despite the biocompatibility of calcium–phosphorus compounds, their application to the implant surface is considered unreliable by dental clinicians and they are still under investigation for biocompatibility, biodegradation, and immunologic response to the wear particles.

Biofunctional proteins and peptides are candidates for the biological linking between the tissue and surface of inserted medical devices. These molecules have the potential to alter a local environment to biologically favorable circumstances, which can be important to patients with systemic metabolic diseases. There are supposedly two categories of the aforementioned molecules involved in the healing of bone surrounding the implants, namely adhesion molecules and cytokines.[27,47,103] Fibronectin and vitronectin are ECMs for osteogenic cell adhesion, which is the first step for osteogenesis, or bone healing. ECMs are substituted for plasma proteins, which play an important role in blood clotting. Initially, the plasma proteins cover the implant surface, followed by the ECM. However, treatment of the implant surface with these adhesion proteins or functional peptide derivatives accelerates osseointegration at the bone–implant interface.[27,40,44,45,47] Functional peptides have lower antigenicity and easier applicability than the original proteins.[27] Several cytokines contribute to bone healing around an implant. Particularly, BMPs, a subset of growth factor cytokines, are direct enhancers of bone formation.[40,103,104] Recombinant human BMP-2 (rhBMP-2) has been clinically used for bone regeneration; however, no dental implant using this recombinant protein has yet been applied to patients. Some in vivo studies reported on faster osseointegration at the interface between the bone and rhBMP-2-treated implant surfaces.[105,106] However, biological responses to such cytokines are diverse and sensitive to concentration.[3,107] Certain complications, including osteolysis, are disastrous to both patients and dental clinicians, thus necessitating a functional peptide derivative from the original growth factor to reduce undesirable side effects and increase the clinical applicability.

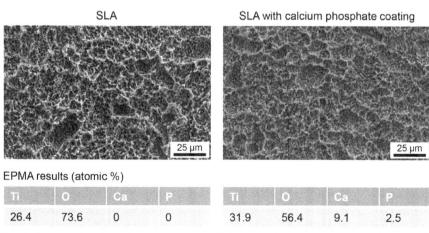

SLA | SLA with calcium phosphate coating

EPMA results (atomic %)

Ti	O	Ca	P	Ti	O	Ca	P
26.4	73.6	0	0	31.9	56.4	9.1	2.5

Fig. 4. Calcium phosphate is nano-coated on SLA surface by ion-bombing. As shown in the results of electron probe microanalysis (EPMA), the surface compositions are different without a large change in microtopography.

The above-mentioned biofunctional molecules are useful for implant surface modification to enhance bone healing. Particularly, adhesion proteins, cytokines, and their derivatives are considered valuable for patients with bone metabolic diseases, because these factors can help to restore compromised bone-healing capacity in the local environment by stimulating osteogenic cell adhesion, osteoblast differentiation, or bone formation activity. At least two problems need to be solved before the clinical use of dental implant surfaces modified with these molecules. The first is the weak binding between the molecules and implant surfaces. Several molecules used for surface functionalization are only physically adsorbed on the surfaces.[108] Physical adsorption can be inadequate for molecule delivery in environments, such as implant surgery that is characterized by high friction between the bone and the functionalized surface.[108] The second is the undesirable side effects of these molecules. Proteins usually exert various effects on a living system. For example, vitronectin is not only beneficial for cell adhesion but also triggers growth factor release by binding to platelets.[40] It is helpful to derive a core amino acid sequence from the original protein for lowering the probability of side effects.[27] However, this core sequence occasionally exerts an unexpected effect than the original protein, thus warranting extensive investigation before considering clinical use.[109]

SUMMARY

The nature of osseointegration is still under investigation. It remains unknown if an implant surface is actively involved in the formation of new bone or if the bone response to this surface is merely a healing process with inflammation. However, topographic, physical, or chemical modifications of the implant surface can change the behavior of cells related to bone healing. Micro-topographical modification is most widely applied to dental implants used in clinics. The resultant surface micro-topography mimics the resorption pits formed by osteoclasts, thus stimulating osteogenic cells to produce bone material. Previously, implant surface treatment at the nano-level was considered ineffective for osteogenesis due to the dimensional aspects of an osteon and incomplete bone ingrowth. Recent evidence suggests that nano-topographical, physical, or molecular changes on the implant surface influence the initial bone response. An implant surface with modified nano-topography has yet to be clinically tested; however, the clinical use of a dental implant has evidence for increased surface hydrophilicity that accelerates the initial bone response. Modified surfaces have been clinically examined in dental implantology with the treatment of some osteogenic elements, such as fluoride anion and calcium–phosphorus compounds. Clinicians have not yet used biofunctional molecules originating from biological adhesion proteins or growth factors. However, these molecules might be bioactive following the treatment of functionalized implant surfaces or useful for improved osseointegration effects in patients with bone metabolic diseases that are currently contraindicated for dental implants. Conjugation problems between biofunctional molecules and implant surfaces and the control of unexpected side effects are under investigation.

CLINICS CARE POINTS

- The sandblasted, large-grit, acid-etched (SLA) surface has shown evidence of success in long-term clinical investigations using implants made of grade 4 commercially pure titanium (cp-Ti). However, the results of SLA surfaces should be evaluated for implants comprising zirconia or materials other than cp-Ti.

- The electrochemically oxidized grade 4 cp-Ti has been shown to be successful in long-term clinical investigations. However, other key factors, including implant design, should be considered as additional factors determining success.
- The use of dental implants modified at the nano-level needs further clinical investigation, despite the use of some physically (hydrophilic surface) or chemically modified surfaces (fluoride-treated and hydroxyapatite-coated surfaces) in dental clinics.

DISCLOSURE

This work was supported by the Korea Medical Device Development Fund grant funded by the Korean government (the Ministry of Science and ICT, the Ministry of Trade, Industry and Energy, the Ministry of Health & Welfare, the Ministry of Food and Drug Safety) (Project number: 1711138190, KMDF_PR_20200901_0105).

REFERENCES

1. Albrektsson T, Branemark PI, Hansson HA, et al. Osseointegrated titanium implants. Requirements for ensuring a long-lasting, direct bone-to-implant anchorage in man. Acta Orthop Scand 1981;52(2):155–70.
2. Souza JCM, Sordi MB, Kanazawa M, et al. Nano-scale modification of titanium implant surfaces to enhance osseointegration. Acta Biomater 2019;94:112–31.
3. Yeo IL. Modifications of dental implant surfaces at the micro- and nano-level for enhanced osseointegration. Materials (Basel) 2019;13(1):89.
4. Almas K, Smith S, Kutkut A. What is the best micro and macro dental implant topography? Dent Clin North Am 2019;63(3):447–60.
5. Rupp F, Liang L, Geis-Gerstorfer J, et al. Surface characteristics of dental implants: a review. Dent Mater 2018;34(1):40–57.
6. Hafezeqoran A, Koodaryan R. Effect of zirconia dental implant surfaces on bone integration: a systematic review and meta-analysis. Biomed Res Int 2017;2017:9246721.
7. Jiang X, Yao Y, Tang W, et al. Design of dental implants at materials level: an overview. J Biomed Mater Res A 2020;108(8):1634–61.
8. Sivaraman K, Chopra A, Narayan AI, et al. Is zirconia a viable alternative to titanium for oral implant? A critical review. J Prosthodont Res 2018;62(2):121–33.
9. Karthigeyan S, Ravindran AJ, Bhat RTR, et al. Surface modification techniques for zirconia-based bioceramics: a review. J Pharm Bioallied Sci 2019;11(Suppl 2):S131–4.
10. Schunemann FH, Galarraga-Vinueza ME, Magini R, et al. Zirconia surface modifications for implant dentistry. Mater Sci Eng C Mater Biol Appl 2019;98:1294–305.
11. Liu Y, Bao C, Wismeijer D, et al. The physicochemical/biological properties of porous tantalum and the potential surface modification techniques to improve its clinical application in dental implantology. Mater Sci Eng C Mater Biol Appl 2015;49:323–9.
12. Jemt T. Implant survival in the edentulous jaw-30 years of experience. Part I: a retro-prospective multivariate regression analysis of overall implant failure in 4,585 consecutively treated arches. Int J Prosthodont 2018;31(5):425–35.
13. Jemt T. Implant survival in the edentulous jaw: 30 years of experience. Part II: A retro-prospective multivariate regression analysis related to treated arch and implant surface roughness. Int J Prosthodont 2018;31(6):531–9.

14. Jemt T. Implant survival in the partially edentulous Jaw- 30 years of experience. Part III: a retro-prospective multivariate regression analysis on overall implant failures in 2,915 consecutively treated arches. Int J Prosthodont 2019;32(1): 36–44.

15. Lee JH, Kim JC, Kim HY, et al. Influence of connections and surfaces of dental implants on marginal bone loss: a retrospective study over 7 to 19 years. Int J Oral Maxillofac Implants 2020;35(6):1195–202.

16. Haas R, Mensdorff-Pouilly N, Mailath G, et al. Survival of 1,920 IMZ implants followed for up to 100 months. Int J Oral Maxillofac Implants 1996;11(5):581–8.

17. Hobo S. Osseointegration and occlusal rehabilitation. (IL): Quintessence Publishing; 1989.

18. Bellows CG, Heersche JN, Aubin JE. The effects of fluoride on osteoblast progenitors in vitro. J Bone Miner Res 1990;5(Suppl 1):S101–5.

19. Kassem M, Mosekilde L, Eriksen EF. Effects of fluoride on human bone cells in vitro: differences in responsiveness between stromal osteoblast precursors and mature osteoblasts. Eur J Endocrinol 1994;130(4):381–6.

20. Rupp F, Scheideler L, Olshanska N, et al. Enhancing surface free energy and hydrophilicity through chemical modification of microstructured titanium implant surfaces. J Biomed Mater Res A 2006;76(2):323–34.

21. Rupp F, Scheideler L, Rehbein D, et al. Roughness induced dynamic changes of wettability of acid etched titanium implant modifications. Biomaterials 2004; 25(7–8):1429–38.

22. Schwartz Z, Boyan BD. Underlying mechanisms at the bone-biomaterial interface. J Cell Biochem 1994;56(3):340–7.

23. Albrektsson T. Healing of bone graft: in vivo studies of tissue reactions at autografting of bone in the rabbit tibia. Thesis; 1979.

24. Maggiano IS, Maggiano CM, Clement JG, et al. Three-dimensional reconstruction of Haversian systems in human cortical bone using synchrotron radiation-based micro-CT: morphology and quantification of branching and transverse connections across age. J Anat 2016;228(5):719–32.

25. Wennerberg A, Albrektsson T. On implant surfaces: a review of current knowledge and opinions. Int J Oral Maxillofac Implants 2010;25(1):63–74.

26. Coelho PG, Jimbo R, Tovar N, et al. Osseointegration: hierarchical designing encompassing the macrometer, micrometer, and nanometer length scales. Dent Mater 2015;31(1):37–52.

27. Yeo IS, Min SK, Kang HK, et al. Identification of a bioactive core sequence from human laminin and its applicability to tissue engineering. Biomaterials 2015;73: 96–109.

28. Choi JY, Kim S, Jo SB, et al. A laminin-211-derived bioactive peptide promotes the osseointegration of a sandblasted, large-grit, acid-etched titanium implant. J Biomed Mater Res A 2020;108(5):1214–22.

29. Lee JB, Jo YH, Choi JY, et al. The effect of ultraviolet photofunctionalization on a titanium dental implant with machined surface: An in vitro and in vivo study. Materials (Basel) 2019;12(13):2078.

30. Kwon TK, Choi JY, Park JI, et al. A clue to the existence of bonding between bone and implant surface: an in vivo study. Materials (Basel) 2019;12(7):1187.

31. Gittens RA, Olivares-Navarrete R, Cheng A, et al. The roles of titanium surface micro/nanotopography and wettability on the differential response of human osteoblast lineage cells. Acta Biomater 2013;9(4):6268–77.

32. Choi JY, Albrektsson T, Jeon YJ, et al. Osteogenic cell behavior on titanium surfaces in hard tissue. J Clin Med 2019;8(5):604.

33. Andrukhov O, Huber R, Shi B, et al. Proliferation, behavior, and differentiation of osteoblasts on surfaces of different microroughness. Dent Mater 2016;32(11):1374–84.

34. Albrektsson T, Jemt T, Molne J, et al. On inflammation-immunological balance theory-A critical apprehension of disease concepts around implants: mucositis and marginal bone loss may represent normal conditions and not necessarily a state of disease. Clin Implant Dent Relat Res 2019;21(1):183–9.

35. Hashemi Astaneh S, Faverani LP, Sukotjo C, et al. Atomic layer deposition on dental materials: processing conditions and surface functionalization to improve physical, chemical, and clinical properties - A review. Acta Biomater 2021;121:103–18.

36. Makowiecki A, Hadzik J, Blaszczyszyn A, et al. An evaluation of superhydrophilic surfaces of dental implants - a systematic review and meta-analysis. BMC Oral Health 2019;19(1):79.

37. Kellesarian SV, Malignaggi VR, Kellesarian TV, et al. Does incorporating collagen and chondroitin sulfate matrix in implant surfaces enhance osseointegration? A systematic review and meta-analysis. Int J Oral Maxillofac Surg 2018;47(2):241–51.

38. Kim JJ, Lee JH, Kim JC, et al. Biological responses to the transitional area of dental implants: material- and structure-dependent responses of peri-implant tissue to abutments. Materials (Basel) 2019;13(1):72.

39. Perez RA, Seo SJ, Won JE, et al. Therapeutically relevant aspects in bone repair and regeneration. Mater Today 2015;18(10):573–89.

40. Terheyden H, Lang NP, Bierbaum S, et al. Osseointegration–communication of cells. Clin Oral Implants Res 2012;23(10):1127–35.

41. Yeo I-S. Surface modification of dental biomaterials for controlling bone response. In: Piattelli A, editor. Bone response to dental implant materials. Duxford: Woodhead Publishing; 2017. p. 43–64.

42. Bosch-Rue E, Diez-Tercero L, Giordano-Kelhoffer B, et al. Biological roles and delivery strategies for ions to promote osteogenic induction. Front Cell Dev Biol 2020;8:614545.

43. Vroman L, Adams AL, Fischer GC, et al. Interaction of high molecular weight kininogen, factor XII, and fibrinogen in plasma at interfaces. Blood 1980;55(1):156–9.

44. Anderson JM, Rodriguez A, Chang DT. Foreign body reaction to biomaterials. Semin Immunol 2008;20(2):86–100.

45. McNally AK, Jones JA, Macewan SR, et al. Vitronectin is a critical protein adhesion substrate for IL-4-induced foreign body giant cell formation. J Biomed Mater Res A 2008;86(2):535–43.

46. Cherny RC, Honan MA, Thiagarajan P. Site-directed mutagenesis of the arginine-glycine-aspartic acid in vitronectin abolishes cell adhesion. J Biol Chem 1993;268(13):9725–9.

47. Cho CB, Jung SY, Park CY, et al. A vitronectin-derived bioactive peptide improves bone healing capacity of SLA titanium surfaces. Materials (Basel) 2019;12(20):3400.

48. Refai AK, Textor M, Brunette DM, et al. Effect of titanium surface topography on macrophage activation and secretion of proinflammatory cytokines and chemokines. J Biomed Mater Res A 2004;70(2):194–205.

49. Song E, Ouyang N, Horbelt M, et al. Influence of alternatively and classically activated macrophages on fibrogenic activities of human fibroblasts. Cell Immunol 2000;204(1):19–28.

50. Choi JY, Sim JH, Yeo IL. Characteristics of contact and distance osteogenesis around modified implant surfaces in rabbit tibiae. J Periodontal Implant Sci 2017;47(3):182–92.

51. Berglundh T, Abrahamsson I, Lang NP, et al. De novo alveolar bone formation adjacent to endosseous implants. Clin Oral Implants Res 2003;14(3):251–62.

52. Frost HM. A 2003 update of bone physiology and Wolff's Law for clinicians. Angle Orthod 2004;74(1):3–15.

53. Blair HC, Larrouture QC, Li Y, et al. Osteoblast differentiation and bone matrix formation in vivo and in vitro. Tissue Eng B Rev 2017;23(3):268–80.

54. Hardy E, Fernandez-Patron C. Destroy to rebuild: the connection between bone tissue remodeling and matrix metalloproteinases. Front Physiol 2020;11:47.

55. Hefti T, Frischherz M, Spencer ND, et al. A comparison of osteoclast resorption pits on bone with titanium and zirconia surfaces. Biomaterials 2010;31(28): 7321–31.

56. Sims NA, Gooi JH. Bone remodeling: multiple cellular interactions required for coupling of bone formation and resorption. Semin Cell Dev Biol 2008;19(5): 444–51.

57. Gray C, Boyde A, Jones SJ. Topographically induced bone formation in vitro: implications for bone implants and bone grafts. Bone 1996;18(2):115–23.

58. Blanes RJ, Bernard JP, Blanes ZM, et al. A 10-year prospective study of ITI dental implants placed in the posterior region. I: Clinical and radiographic results. Clin Oral Implants Res 2007;18(6):699–706.

59. Kim DM, Badovinac RL, Lorenz RL, et al. A 10-year prospective clinical and radiographic study of one-stage dental implants. Clin Oral Implants Res 2008; 19(3):254–8.

60. Weber HP, Crohin CC, Fiorellini JP. A 5-year prospective clinical and radiographic study of non-submerged dental implants. Clin Oral Implants Res 2000;11(2):144–53.

61. Wennerberg A, Albrektsson T, Johansson C, et al. Experimental study of turned and grit-blasted screw-shaped implants with special emphasis on effects of blasting material and surface topography. Biomaterials 1996;17(1):15–22.

62. Schupbach P, Glauser R, Bauer S. Al_2O_3 particles on titanium dental implant systems following sandblasting and acid-etching process. Int J Biomater 2019;2019:6318429.

63. Chacun D, Lafon A, Courtois N, et al. Histologic and histomorphometric evaluation of new zirconia-based ceramic dental implants: A preclinical study in dogs. Dent Mater 2021;37(9):1377–89.

64. Majhi R, Majhi RK, Garhnayak L, et al. Comparative evaluation of surface-modified zirconia for the growth of bone cells and early osseointegration. J Prosthet Dent 2021;126(1):92 e1–8.

65. Choi JY, Kang SH, Kim HY, et al. Control variable implants improve interpretation of surface modification and implant design effects on early bone responses: an in vivo study. Int J Oral Maxillofac Implants 2018;33(5):1033–40.

66. Lee HJ, Yang IH, Kim SK, et al. In vivo comparison between the effects of chemically modified hydrophilic and anodically oxidized titanium surfaces on initial bone healing. J Periodontal Implant Sci 2015;45(3):94–100.

67. Cooper LF. A role for surface topography in creating and maintaining bone at titanium endosseous implants. J Prosthet Dent 2000;84(5):522–34.

68. Momesso GAC, Santos AMS, Fonseca ESJM, et al. Comparison between plasma electrolytic oxidation coating and sandblasted acid-etched surface

treatment: histometric, tomographic, and expression levels of osteoclastogenic factors in osteoporotic rats. Materials (Basel) 2020;13(7):1604.

69. Ernst S, Stubinger S, Schupbach P, et al. Comparison of two dental implant surface modifications on implants with same macrodesign: an experimental study in the pelvic sheep model. Clin Oral Implants Res 2015;26(8):898–908.

70. Bonfante EA, Janal MN, Granato R, et al. Buccal and lingual bone level alterations after immediate implantation of four implant surfaces: a study in dogs. Clin Oral Implants Res 2013;24(12):1375–80.

71. Koh JW, Kim YS, Yang JH, et al. Effects of a calcium phosphate-coated and anodized titanium surface on early bone response. Int J Oral Maxillofac Implants 2013;28(3):790–7.

72. Rossi F, Lang NP, Ricci E, et al. Long-term follow-up of single crowns supported by short, moderately rough implants-A prospective 10-year cohort study. Clin Oral Implants Res 2018;29(12):1212–9.

73. van Velzen FJ, Ofec R, Schulten EA, et al. 10-year survival rate and the incidence of peri-implant disease of 374 titanium dental implants with a SLA surface: a prospective cohort study in 177 fully and partially edentulous patients. Clin Oral Implants Res 2015;26(10):1121–8.

74. Roccuzzo M, Bonino L, Dalmasso P, et al. Long-term results of a three arms prospective cohort study on implants in periodontally compromised patients: 10-year data around sandblasted and acid-etched (SLA) surface. Clin Oral Implants Res 2014;25(10):1105–12.

75. Degidi M, Nardi D, Piattelli A. 10-year follow-up of immediately loaded implants with TiUnite porous anodized surface. Clin Implant Dent Relat Res 2012;14(6):828–38.

76. Jemt T. Implant survival in the posterior partially edentulous arch-30 years of experience. Part IV: a retro-prospective multivariable regression analysis on implant failures related to arch and implant surface. Int J Prosthodont 2019;32(2):143–52.

77. Chrcanovic BR, Albrektsson T, Wennerberg A. Turned versus anodised dental implants: a meta-analysis. J Oral Rehabil 2016;43(9):716–28.

78. Rice JM, Hunt JA, Gallagher JA, et al. Quantitative assessment of the response of primary derived human osteoblasts and macrophages to a range of nanotopography surfaces in a single culture model in vitro. Biomaterials 2003;24(26):4799–818.

79. Wennerberg A, Albrektsson T. Suggested guidelines for the topographic evaluation of implant surfaces. Int J Oral Maxillofac Implants 2000;15(3):331–44.

80. Kunrath MF, Leal BF, Hubler R, et al. Antibacterial potential associated with drug-delivery built TiO_2 nanotubes in biomedical implants. AMB Express 2019;9(1):51.

81. Miao X, Wang D, Xu L, et al. The response of human osteoblasts, epithelial cells, fibroblasts, macrophages and oral bacteria to nanostructured titanium surfaces: a systematic study. Int J Nanomedicine 2017;12:1415–30.

82. Shin YC, Pang KM, Han DW, et al. Enhanced osteogenic differentiation of human mesenchymal stem cells on Ti surfaces with electrochemical nanopattern formation. Mater Sci Eng C Mater Biol Appl 2019;99:1174–81.

83. Liu H, Webster TJ. Nanomedicine for implants: a review of studies and necessary experimental tools. Biomaterials 2007;28(2):354–69.

84. Li T, Gulati K, Wang N, et al. Understanding and augmenting the stability of therapeutic nanotubes on anodized titanium implants. Mater Sci Eng C Mater Biol Appl 2018;88:182–95.

85. Ahn TK, Lee DH, Kim TS, et al. Modification of titanium implant and titanium dioxide for bone tissue engineering. Adv Exp Med Biol 2018;1077:355–68.

86. Awad NK, Edwards SL, Morsi YS. A review of TiO_2 NTs on Ti metal: electrochemical synthesis, functionalization and potential use as bone implants. Mater Sci Eng C Mater Biol Appl 2017;76:1401–12.

87. Park J, Bauer S, Schlegel KA, et al. TiO_2 nanotube surfaces: 15 nm–an optimal length scale of surface topography for cell adhesion and differentiation. Small 2009;5(6):666–71.

88. Oh S, Brammer KS, Li YS, et al. Stem cell fate dictated solely by altered nanotube dimension. Proc Natl Acad Sci U S A 2009;106(7):2130–5.

89. Nicolau P, Guerra F, Reis R, et al. 10-year outcomes with immediate and early loaded implants with a chemically modified SLA surface. Quintessence Int 2019;50(2):114–24.

90. Morra M, Cassinelli C, Bruzzone G, et al. Surface chemistry effects of topographic modification of titanium dental implant surfaces: 1. Surface analysis. Int J Oral Maxillofac Implants 2003;18(1):40–5.

91. Puisys A, Schlee M, Linkevicius T, et al. Photo-activated implants: a triple-blinded, split-mouth, randomized controlled clinical trial on the resistance to removal torque at various healing intervals. Clin Oral Investig 2020;24(5):1789–99.

92. Ogawa T. Ultraviolet photofunctionalization of titanium implants. Int J Oral Maxillofac Implants 2014;29(1):e95–102.

93. Hirota M, Ozawa T, Iwai T, et al. Effect of photofunctionalization on early implant failure. Int J Oral Maxillofac Implants 2018;33(5):1098–102.

94. Ellingsen JE, Thomsen P, Lyngstadaas SP. Advances in dental implant materials and tissue regeneration. Periodontol 2000 2006;41:136–56.

95. Windael S, Vervaeke S, Wijnen L, et al. Ten-year follow-up of dental implants used for immediate loading in the edentulous mandible: a prospective clinical study. Clin Implant Dent Relat Res 2018;20(4):515–21.

96. Donati M, Ekestubbe A, Lindhe J, et al. Marginal bone loss at implants with different surface characteristics - A 20-year follow-up of a randomized controlled clinical trial. Clin Oral Implants Res 2018;29(5):480–7.

97. Sun L, Berndt CC, Gross KA, et al. Material fundamentals and clinical performance of plasma-sprayed hydroxyapatite coatings: a review. J Biomed Mater Res 2001;58(5):570–92.

98. Um SH, Lee J, Song IS, et al. Regulation of cell locomotion by nanosecond-laser-induced hydroxyapatite patterning. Bioact Mater 2021;6(10):3608–19.

99. Safi IN, Hussein BMA, Aljudy HJ, et al. Effects of long durations of RF-magnetron sputtering deposition of hydroxyapatite on titanium dental implants. Eur J Den 2021;15(3):440–7.

100. Lopez-Valverde N, Flores-Fraile J, Ramirez JM, et al. Bioactive surfaces vs. conventional surfaces in titanium dental implants: a comparative systematic review. J Clin Med 2020;9(7):2047.

101. Artzi Z, Carmeli G, Kozlovsky A. A distinguishable observation between survival and success rate outcome of hydroxyapatite-coated implants in 5-10 years in function. Clin Oral Implants Res 2006;17(1):85–93.

102. Alsabeeha NH, Ma S, Atieh MA. Hydroxyapatite-coated oral implants: a systematic review and meta-analysis. Int J Oral Maxillofac Implants 2012;27(5):1123–30.

103. Song R, Wang D, Zeng R, et al. Synergistic effects of fibroblast growth factor-2 and bone morphogenetic protein-2 on bone induction. Mol Med Rep 2017;16(4): 4483–92.

104. Rogers MB, Shah TA, Shaikh NN. Turning bone morphogenetic protein 2 (BMP2) on and off in mesenchymal cells. J Cell Biochem 2015;116(10):2127–38.

105. Kim S, Park C, Moon BS, et al. Enhancement of osseointegration by direct coating of rhBMP-2 on target-ion induced plasma sputtering treated SLA surface for dental application. J Biomater Appl 2017;31(6):807–18.

106. Zhang Y, Hu L, Lin M, et al. RhBMP-2-Loaded PLGA/titanium nanotube delivery system synergistically enhances osseointegration. ACS Omega 2021;6(25): 16364–72.

107. De Stefano FA, Elarjani T, Burks JD, et al. Dose adjustment associated complications of bone morphogenetic protein: a longitudinal assessment. World Neurosurg 2021;S1878-8750(21):01330–9. https://doi.org/10.1016/j.wneu.2021. 08.142.

108. Stewart C, Akhavan B, Wise SG, et al. A review of biomimetic surface functionalization for bone-integrating orthopedic implants: Mechanisms, current approaches, and future directions. Prog Mater Sci 2019;106:100588.

109. Min SK, Kang HK, Jung SY, et al. A vitronectin-derived peptide reverses ovariectomy-induced bone loss via regulation of osteoblast and osteoclast differentiation. Cell Death Differ 2018;25(2):268–81.

Regenerating the Dental Pulp–Scaffold Materials and Approaches

Diana Gabriela Soares, DDS, MSc, PhD[a], Vinicius Rosa, DDS, MSc, PhD[b],*

KEYWORDS

- Tissue engineering • Odontoblastic differentiation • Dentin formation • 3D printing
- Bioactive materials • Growth factors

KEY POINTS

- Emerging technologies (bioactive scaffolds, 3-dimensional printing, cell sheets) to promote the regeneration of functional dental pulp.
- Advanced materials and strategies to manufacture scaffolds with enhanced bioactivity and regenerative potential.
- Cell-homing and cell-free strategies that allow odontoblastic differentiation and dental pulp regeneration.

INTRODUCTION

Dental pulp has sensorial, defensive, and proprioceptive functions. After severe tooth trauma or exposure to bacterial infection, the pulp is likely to become necrotic, requiring its complete removal and replacement with materials that aim to seal the root space and avoid further infection. The absence of vital pulp tissue eradicates the humoral and cellular defenses mediated by the immune system, and the nutritive and sensorial functions essential for tooth homeostasis, protection, and root development.

The traditional vital pulp therapy is a reparative strategy, which involves the application of alkaline cements on the injured pulp to promote an inflammatory reaction that can trigger resident cells present in the viable pulp tissue to produce a dentinal barrier via dystrophic calcification.[1,2] However, the heterogenicity of the dentinal barrier can compromise pulp sealing, making the tissue more susceptible to recurrent infections. Moreover, vital pulp therapy is less effective in older patients or in areas where the pulp

[a] Department of Operative Dentistry, Endodontics and Dental Materials, São Paulo University – USP, Bauru School of Dentistry, Dr. Octavio Pinheiro Brizola, 9-75, Bauru, Sao Paulo 17012-901, Brazil; [b] Faculty of Dentistry, National University of Singapore, 9 Lower Kent Ridge Road, Level 10, Singapore 119085, Singapore
* Corresponding author.
E-mail addresses: soares.dg@usp.br (D.G.S.); vini@nus.edu.sg (V.R.)

Dent Clin N Am 66 (2022) 643–657
https://doi.org/10.1016/j.cden.2022.05.010
0011-8532/22/© 2022 Elsevier Inc. All rights reserved.
dental.theclinics.com

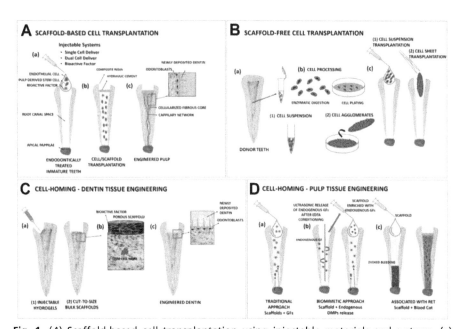

Fig. 1. (*A*) Scaffold-based cell transplantation using injectable materials and systems. (a) Injectable scaffolds are implanted along with cells and/or bioactive factors in the root canal space of endodontically treated (disinfected) teeth. (b) The transplanted teeth are sealed with hydraulic cement and composite resin to generate (c) engineered pulp tissue containing a cellularized fibrous core, with odontoblast-like cells lining the native dentin and extended cytoplasmatic prolongments inside the newly deposited dentin. The establishment of a capillary network from apical tissues is desirable. (*B*) Scaffold-free cell transplantation proposed by in vivo clinical trials. (a) A donor tooth from the same patient (deciduous tooth or third molar) is used as a source for progenitor cells that are (b) processed and cultured in vitro to obtain cell suspensions or cell agglomerates. (c) These cultured cells are transplanted into endodontically treated (disinfected) teeth to create engineered dental pulp. (*C*) Cell-homing strategies for dentin tissue engineering. (a) Injectable hydrogels or cut-to-size bulk scaffolds made of synthetic natural polymers are used as direct pulp capping agents. (b) A porous structure is desirable, and biomaterials are associated with bioactive factors to induce resident pulp cell chemotaxis, which would result in the engineered dentin (c) containing odontoblast-like cells and newly deposited dentin to seal pulp exposure. (*D*) Cell-homing strategies for dental pulp tissue engineering. (a) The traditional approach uses injectable scaffolds (usually collagen) enriched with recombinant growth factors. (b) The biomimetic approach takes advantage of endogenous growth factors (dentin matrix proteins) released by EDTA treatment and ultrasonic irrigation, which are later incorporated into the scaffold. (c) The association of a naturally derived scaffold with the evoked bleeding technique is a current strategy that aims to achieve more reliable pulp-like regeneration by using the regenerative endodontic treatment strategy.

exposure is deemed too large. Finally, calcium hydroxide, which is often used to promote the formation of a calcified barrier, can increase the chances of root fracture over time.[3]

In early 2000s, a new strategy for managing root canals based on provoking bleeding into the canal after disinfection procedures emerged.[4] The evoked bleeding technique is based on the over instrumentation of apical tissue to produce a blood clot, which can home stem cells and growth factors from apical tissues, to promote tooth revitalization, to narrow the root apex, and to increase the dentinal wall thickness

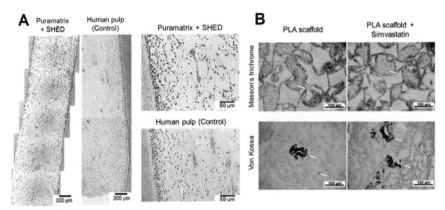

Fig. 2. (*A*) In vivo dental pulp tissue engineering. The injection of Puramatrix (Corning, USA) mixed with SHED has allowed for the formation of a vascularized connective tissue within the full-length human root canals occupied the full extension of the root canal.[30]. (*B*) Simvastatin and nanofibrous poly(ʟ-lactic acid) scaffolds loaded with DPSC promote the odontogenic differentiation and the regeneration of a pulp-like tissue in vivo. The formation of a collagen-rich matrix surrounded by cells was confirmed by Masson's trichrome staining while and the Von Kossa revealed mineralized structures in the scaffold's macropores dental pulp cells.[53]

and root length.[4,5] In fact, immature teeth treated with regenerative endodontic treatment have experienced significant increases root length and width (14% and 28%) when compared with teeth where apexification was induced by mineral trioxide aggregate (MTA; 6% and 0%) or calcium hydroxide (0.4% and 1.5%).[6] These seem to be derived from a reparative event, in which the soft tissue resembles the periodontal ligament alongside cementum/bone-like tissue deposition into the root canal space and on the dentin walls.[7,8] Moreover, the conditioning agent used to treat the dentin before the bleeding is evoked (such as ethylenediaminetetraacetic acid [EDTA]) can promote the release of biomolecules, noncollagenous proteins, growth factors, and glycosaminoglycans from the dentin matrix, which modulate important biological processes involved in the revascularization and pulp regeneration.[9,10] For instance, cell migration and proliferation are stimulated by transforming growth factor β1 (TGF-β1) and fibroblast growth factors 2, whereas bone morphogenetic proteins 2 (BMP-2) promotes odontoblastic differentiation and dentinogenesis.[11] Moreover, the blood clot acts as a natural scaffold formed by a meshwork of fibrin strands containing platelets, endothelial cells, ions and enzymes that induce cell migration and differentiation and support tissue formation and revascularization.[4,12]

Ever since, the regenerative endodontic treatment has become a clinical reality for the management of necrotic and irreversible pulpitis, with success rates varying from 81% to 96% for immature permanent teeth after at least 1-year follow-up.[13,14] Long-term regenerative endodontic treatment outcomes may include obliteration of the root canal, tooth discoloration, and persistent bacterial infection, whereas further root development is not always achieved.[13,14]

When vital pulp therapy regenerative endodontic treatment or strategies fail, the pulp is replaced by (mostly inert) materials. Endodontically treated teeth become more susceptible to recurrent infections and trauma. This is even more concerning in immature teeth because incomplete root formation results in fragile teeth more susceptible to catastrophic failure.[15] Hence, further development of strategies and technologies to promote the regeneration of functional dental pulp is of high interest.

The developments in tissue engineering have inspired and enabled remarkable achievements toward the regeneration of functional dental pulp for the preservation and healthy development of injured teeth.[16] This can be accomplished through several approaches but some of them are attracting more attention due to their versatility and promising (in vitro and in vivo) data such as (1) multifunctional scaffolds and biomaterials to modulate cell proliferation and differentiation toward pulp–dentin complex regeneration; (2) biomimetic approaches with tailor-made scaffolds to mimic preexisting environmental, mechanical, and biochemical cues to promote specific cell–matrix interactions[17–19]; and (3) scaffold-free strategies using cell agglomerates with intense regenerative potential.[20–22] The objective of this review is to highlight and discuss recent developments, novel strategies, and emerging technologies in dental pulp tissue engineering (**Fig. 1**).

DENTAL PULP REGENERATION USING SCAFFOLD-BASED AND CELL TRANSPLANTATION TECHNOLOGIES

Cell-based pulp tissue engineering requires the orchestration of cells, scaffolds, and signaling pathways.[23–25] In several cell-based strategies, stem cells are seeded in scaffolds that serve as frameworks for tissue ingrowth (examples of commonly used polymers for scaffold fabrication are shown in **Table 1**[18]). Stem cells from deciduous (SHED) or permanent teeth dental pulp stem cells (DPSC) offer important advantages. For instance, DPSC express several mesenchymal stem cell markers, and their gene profile is analogous to bone marrow stem cells on approximately 4400 genes.[26–28] They can be obtained from extracted teeth, which is a much simpler procedure than bone marrow aspiration. Finally, stem cells from dental pulp have an ectomesodermic origin and can differentiate into neurons, which can contribute to the regeneration of functional and sensitive dental pulp.[29] Three cell-based strategies with high potential for clinical translation have emerged, namely injectable scaffolds, microspheres systems to provide carrier and sustained release systems, and decellularized tissues, which are inserted into a biomimetic approach.

Hydrogel scaffolds have a promising clinical translation appeal for pulp regeneration because they can be inserted into the narrow and irregular architecture of root canals in liquid form before gelation.[30] The hydrogels can be functionalized with growth factors to trigger and augment cell functions. However, biofunctionalization can increase the costs of production and the risks of immunogenicity.

Self-assembly peptide (SAP) hydrogels present good injectability, allow for functional domains such as arginine, glycine, and aspartate (RGD) domain, and may present a nanoarchitecture that mimics the natural extracellular matrix. The SAP hydrogels have been explored as scaffolds and carriers for pulp-derived cells, endothelial cells, and growth factors. Injectable SAP hydrogels combined with SHED have promoted the establishment of pulp-like tissue in the full length of the root canal implanted in an animal model. Notably, the tissue formed with SAP/SHED secreted new dentin along the walls similarly to the pulp formed with recombinant type I collagen hydrogel.[30] The SAP hydrogels can also serve as effective cell carriers and have been shown to improve the revascularization of engineered dental pulps when used to promote the dual-cell delivery system of DPSC associated with endothelial cells.[31] Despite their promising potential for pulp regeneration, SAP hydrogels are mostly inert and do not trigger or enhance odontoblastic differentiation (**Fig. 2**).[30]

Hydrogels based on gelatin methacrylate (GelMA) have gained popularity due to their low production costs, low immunogenicity, and structural similarities with the natural extracellular matrix provided by gelatin. GelMA incorporates approximately 5% of

Table 1
Pulp regeneration

Polymers for Scaffold Production	Relevant Characteristics for Dental Pulp Regeneration		
Collagen[30,66,69]	Biocompatibility and bioactivity, promotes cell migration and growth	Allows for the incorporation of bioactive materials	Physical and mechanical properties can be fined tuned via chemical cross-linking	Cross-linking procedures can compromise cell survival
Fibrin[70–72]	Natural biomaterial, good biocompatibility and cell adhesion	Enriches the microenvironment with growth factors and provides a suitable environment for angiogenesis	Mechanical properties can be improved with the addition of hyaluronic acid or β-tricalcium phosphate	Has low stiffness and degrades fast
Polycaprolactone[52,65]	High biocompatibility and acceptable mechanical properties	Very low degradation rate and lacks cell recognition sites	Can be modified with hydroxyapatite and mineral trioxide aggregate to increase its bioactivity and degradation rate	Rigid, cannot be injected but allows for the fabrication of 3-dimensional printed scaffolds
Other synthetic polymers (polyglycolic acid, polylactide-Co-glycolide, polylactic acid)[11,16]	High biocompatibility and proven track record in pulp regeneration	Allow for the incorporation of biomolecules and growth factors to increase biological responses	Physical and mechanical properties can be adjusted by changes in monomers molecular weight/ratio and crystallinity	Rigid, cannot be injected, can be easily cast in dentin slices, may require organic solvents for fabrication

methacrylic anhydride, which does not interfere with biological functions or biologically active motifs, whereas the mechanical properties can be adjusted. The potential of GelMA to regenerate dental pulp has been observed in root canals (6 mm length) injected with GelMA-containing DPSC and endothelial cells. In this experiment, a pulp-like tissue containing an organized and functional vascular network was formed. The tissues formed also presented odontoblast-like cells lining the dentin surface, featuring cellular extensions into dentin tubules and new dentin deposition.[32] Another proposed strategy merges GelMA and microfluidic technology to create a vascularized core inside the root canal. Here, a sacrificial fiber is populated by endothelial cells to home cells from apical tissues. This strategy resulted in angiogenic sprouting within 7 days in vitro.[33] Further developments in GelMA composition include the incorporation of photoinitiators to promote faster polymerization of this hydrogel. This has allowed for the encapsulation of dental pulp cells, odontoblastic differentiation, and the fabrication of vascularized constructs in GelMA with predefined spatial arrangements.[34,35] GelMA can be further modified with growth factors and compounds to provide angiogenic, chemotactic, osteoblastic, and odontoblastic differention potential, as well as anti-inflammatory properties.[34,36] The encapsulation of antibiotics and other compounds (eg, nanofibers and hollow nanotubes) in GelMA can create cell-friendly platforms for infection ablation and tissue regeneration.[37,38]

Microspheres have been proposed for pulp tissue engineering as injectable systems able to act as a cell carrier (such as a scaffold) and promote the delivery of drug and growth factors. Poly(L-lactic acid) (PLLA) microspheres present promising nanoscale ($\sim$160 nm diameter) topography-mimicking natural collagen architecture that may facilitate cell adhesion, proliferation, and differentiation. This system has been used to regenerate the pulp of endodontically treated first molars in mice. The DPSC encapsulated in hollow nanofibrous-PLLA microspheres regenerated pulp-like tissue intimately integrated to the native dentin after 4 weeks.[39] Microspheres can also be used as a dual delivery system for sustained release of compounds. Promising results have been observed in heparin-conjugated gelatin nanospheres loaded with both DPSC and vascular endothelial growth factor (VEGF) that regenerated pulp-like tissue filling 9 mm from the apical to the coronal third of human premolar root canals (total root length of 13 mm, **Fig. 3**). The tissue formed contained many blood vessels and odontoblast-like cells aligned with the existing tubular root dentin.[40] The potential of microspheres to promote rapid vascularization of engineered pulp tissue has been achieved through the encapsulation of human platelet lysate, a natural-derived pool of multiple growth factors, into a GelMA microspheres system. This system has achieved sustained release of growth factors for 28 days and modulated DPSC migration and angiogenesis in vitro. It has also led to the formation of pulp-like tissue in human tooth fragments implanted in vivo. The tissues formed were rich in the extracellular matrix, the cells lining the blood vessels were positive for CD-31 positive cells, and the odontoblast-like cells at the dentin wall presented a positive expression of dentin matrix acidic phosphoprotein 1 (DMP-1).[41]

A decellularized dental pulp extracellular matrix (dECM) has been proposed to create biomimetic multifunctional hydrogels for pulp–dentin complex regeneration. Decellularization results in a structure that retains the native biological molecules, creating a microenvironment that can trigger, modulate, and enhance cellular adhesion, proliferation, migration, and differentiation.[42,43] Furthermore, the removal of the cellular components reduces the risk of adverse immune responses.[41] The dECM has been combined with hydrogel to produce scaffolds with bioacte potential that have regenerated a vascularized pulp-like tissue in human tooth slices implanted in animal models. Despite the ease of manufacturing and clinical appeal due to its

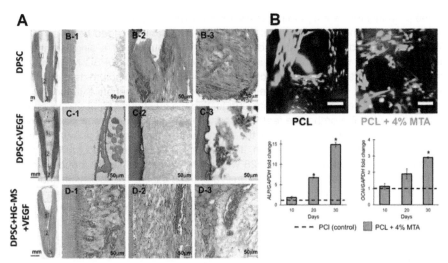

Fig. 3. The addition of growth factors and inorganic compounds can increase the bioactivity of scaffolds used for pulp regeneration. (A) Histologic analysis of regenerated pulp-like tissues in the full-length root canal after in vivo implantation with DPSC, DPSC combined with VEGF or DPSC combined with hierarchical microsphere loaded with VEGF. The latter has enabled the regeneration of a pulp-like tissue that occupied almost the totality of the root canal space and has promoted the differentiation of DPSC into odontoblast-like cells lining the root dentin.[40] (B) The bioactivity of the 3D printed polycaprolactone (PCL) scaffold can be enhanced by the addition of 4% of mineral trioxide aggregate to increase the expression of genes commonly associated with cells able to secret mineralized deposits (ALP and OCN, * means p<0.05).[52]

injectability potential, the limited amount of pulp tissue available in human teeth for decellularization limits this promising technique.[44] Therefore, xenogenic pulp tissues obtained from other mammals have been explored to create dECM-based hydrogels for pulp regeneration.[45] Chemical decellularization of rat dental pulp resulted in a scaffold with a well-preserved collagen fiber network in the entire matrix, with weak immunoreactivity to collagen type I and III antigens. Notably, the dECM scaffold allowed DPSC to proliferate and induced higher expressions of dentin sialophosphoprotein (DSPP), DMP-1, VEGF-A, and vascular endothelial growth factor receptor 2 after 14 days in culture.[46] Swine dental pulp tissues have been found to be promising alternatives for solving the low dECM production yield. On decellularization, the scaffold conserved collagen I throughout the matrix, whereas Von Willebrand factor was observed around the blood vessels, and dentin sialoprotein (DSP) and DMP-1 were labeled in the tissue periphery near the dentinal walls.[46] The implantation of dECM in beagle dogs' molars and premolars with open apices revealed cellular infiltration from the apex up to the pulp chambers 8 weeks after the implantation. The dECM created a promising environment for the recruitment of vascular cells and promoted the differentiation of cells from the periapical tissues to produce pulp-like tissue with positive expression for DSP.[47] Although dECM has promising potential to regenerate vascularized pulp-like tissues, its production often involves the use of detergents to promote the decellularization. Unfortunately, these compounds can alter, remove, or even degrade important components present in the extracellular matrix, such as laminin, which is critical for odontoblast differentiation and DSP expression regulation.[48]

The potential for dental pulp regeneration goes beyond preclinical models and has been asserted in humans. A clinical study included 5 subjects aged between 20 and 55 years who had been diagnosed with irreversible pulpitis of a single root canal and were treated with autologous implantation of "mobilized" DPSC retrieved from sound third molars and seeded in clinical grade atelocollagen scaffolds. Four weeks after the scaffold implantation, the patients evolved from negative to positive responses during the electric pulp tests, suggesting the reestablishment of reinnervated pulp tissue. After 6 months, the teeth treated with scaffolds presented magnetic resonance imaging parameters such as the sound (untreated) controls, indicating complete pulp regeneration. In addition, the radiographs and cone beam computed tomography analyses performed at 28 weeks showed lateral dentin deposition and obliteration of the enlarged apical portion in 3 of the 5 cases. These clinical and imaging data are robust evidence that scaffolds and dental stem cells can regenerate functional pulp tissue able to transmit sensory signals and recover vascular supply in clinical scenarios.[49]

Cell-Homing and Scaffold-Free Technologies for Pulp–Dentin Complex Regeneration

In cell-homing strategies, scaffolds (bioactive or saturated with growth factors) are inserted or injected into root canals to induce the migration of endogenous stem/progenitor cells from periapical tissues or remaining dental pulp to promote further proliferation and differentiation.[50] Many cut-to-size bulk scaffolds, injectable hydrogels, and biopolymers have been identified as potential candidates to mimic pulp and the dentin extracellular matrix and offer recognition sites for cells, thus enhancing their differentiation potential.[51,52] Scaffolds used in cell-homing strategies need to present interconnected macro-porous networks to allow cell–cell interactions, tissue ingrowth, and adequate vascularization.[18,38,51–53] Controlling all spatial parameters is very challenging because changes in input parameters (eg, pore size or scaffold composition) may significantly influence the overall characteristics and performance of the scaffold (eg, bioactivity and the degradation rate).[52] Similarly, the incorporation of bioactive cues, such as growth factors or bioactive materials, can improve chemotaxis, cell proliferation and differentiation, and increase mineralization potential.[18,52] For instance, the incorporation of MTA into polycaprolactone (a polymer that degrades slowly) can increase the scaffold degradation rate and promote DPSC differentiation.[52] The incorporation of simvastatin, dexamethasone, vitamin D3, and other pleiotropic molecules at specific bioactive dosages on cell-free scaffolds can modulate chemotaxis, inflammation, and angiogenesis and promote mineralization. The combination of these compounds with mineral phases (eg, calcium aluminate and calcium hydroxide) often results in a synergistic effect in scaffolds that can further boost mineralized matrix deposition.[18,34] One example is a chitosan/calcium hydroxide scaffold doped with simvastatin, which has been shown to modulate dental pulp cells chemotaxis and increase the expression of alkaline phosphatase (ALP), collagen type I alpha 1 chain, DMP-1, and DSPP by DPSC in a 3-dimensional (3D) culture using an artificial pulp chamber model. Implantation of this scaffold seeded with DPSC in an animal model resulted in intense mineralization. The high rate of host cell infiltration toward the scaffold and the mineralization makes this a promising material for cell-homing-based pulp regeneration.[18] Notably, PLLA containing simvastatin recovered the regenerative potential of DPSC under a degenerative inflammatory stimulus. The 'DPSC cultured for 28 days in the simvastatin-containing PLLA scaffolds presented high genetic expressions of DMP-1, DSPP, and BMP-2 and higher angiogenic potential.[53] Another promising multifunctional platform for dentin regeneration is based on the use of a light activated GelMA formulation encapsulated with halloysite clay nanotubes to promote sustained release of dexamethasone. This injectable hydrogel improved the odontogenic differentiation and chemotaxis of SHED in a proinflammatory environment. The hydrogel promoted intense cell recruitment and mineralization after in situ injection in critical defects created in rat calvaria.[34] Collectively, these results confirm that the incorporation of biomolecules and bioactive compounds into polymeric scaffolds can subdue material inertness, promote the recruitment of host cells, and induce their differentiation.[18,34,52,53]

Biomimetic approaches are also viable alternatives for promoting dental pulp and dentin regeneration. Acid-soluble dentin matrix proteins possess high odontogenic and angiogenic potential for inducing dentin bridge deposition in contact with pulp tissue.[54] Notably, dentin-derived BMP-2 is required for SHED odontoblastic differentiation because these cells express different BMP receptors (BMPR) such as BMPR-IA, BMPR-IB, and BMPR-II.[11] Similarly, odontogenic media containing BMP-4 have been used to derive functional odontoblast-like cells from human-induced pluripotent stem cells reprogrammed from DPSC inducing high genetic expressions of matrix extracellular phosphoglycoprotein, DMP-1, and DSPP and increased mineralization potential.[55] Hence, dentin-derived proteins and other growth factors have great potential to promote odontoblastic differentiation and pulp regeneration.

The potential of biomimetic approaches for pulp regeneration has been shown with a dentin-derived bioink, a printable alginate enriched with the soluble and insoluble fractions of the dentin matrix. This hydrogel significantly increased the genetic expression of Runt-related transcription factor 2 (RUNX2) and ALP content in stem cells from the apical papilla (SCAP) in vitro.[56] The clinical potential of biomimetic approaches has been confirmed in a clinical study where mechanically exposed human pulps (premolars scheduled to be extracted for orthodontic reasons) were treated (pulp capping) with an injectable-treated dentin matrix hydrogel. Histologic analyses performed after 2 months revealed the formation of dentin bridges and almost no inflammatory cell infiltration, confirming the biocompatible character of this material. The teeth treated with the hydrogel presented thick dentin bridges and layers of well-arranged odontoblasts that formed homogenous tubular structures with dentinal tubules. In comparison, teeth treated with Biodentine and MTA presented an osteodentin layer with signs of inflammatory reaction on remnant pulp, denoting a reparative event.[57]

Scaffold-based tissue engineering aims to overcome the limitations of material degradability and the limited spatial distribution of cells within the scaffold. Dental stem cells can be used to produce cellular niches to promote pulp-dentin complex regeneration in scaffold-free and growth factor-free environments. A potential advantage of this strategy is that autologous cell transplantation does not raise ethical concerns. Several commercial entities have partnered with dental clinics worldwide for the isolation and banking of dental stem cells.[25]

The potential of scaffold-free strategies, such as sheet-derived pellets produced from SCAP, to promote dental pulp regeneration has been confirmed by several studies. This scaffold-free system regenerated dental pulp-like tissue and produced a continuous layer of dentine-like tissue of uniform thickness along the walls of root canals implanted for 6 weeks in an animal model.[49] Cell sheets (self-assembled 3D scaffold-free tissues) from human dental pulp cells have also regenerated a highly vascularized pulp-like tissue within the root canal after 3-month and 5-month implantations. The tissue also contained populations of cells in close contact with the dentin wall with positive expression for DSP, which suggests the establishment of an odontoblastic-like layer at the dentin surface of root canals containing scaffold-free engineered tissues.[58]

Another potential route is the use of microtissue spheroids produced with DPSC (combined or not with endothelial cells), which have been found to regenerate pulp-like tissue in root canals implanted in animal models. Notably, the tissue formed presented odontoblast-like cells lining the dentin with projected processes into the dentinal tubules and presented positive expression for nestin and DSP, which are typically expressed in odontoblasts.[59]

A groundbreaking study leveraged a scaffold-free approach to regenerate dental pulp in young subjects (7–12 years old) with traumatized immature incisor teeth, featuring incompletely formed apices. The teeth were treated with autologous SHED agglomerates collected from the patients' deciduous canine teeth. The follow-up revealed that the autologous implantation of SHED created the conditions needed for pulp regeneration and root development. Image reconstructions from microtomographic studies showed normal root length with apical foramen closure being achieved at 12 months, whereas the laser Doppler flowmetry showed an increase in vascular formation in the teeth that received the SHED. The histopathological features of one transplanted tooth denoted regeneration of the whole dental pulp tissue containing an odontoblastic layer, connective tissue, and blood vessels, with cells expressing neuronal markers.[12] These exciting results show that cell-laden tissue engineering strategies for pulp–dentin complex regeneration are a feasible technology with evident clinical potential.

OUTLOOK AND CHALLENGES

The advancements in regenerative strategies, technology, and material sciences have enabled remarkable achievements in dental pulp tissue engineering. Today, clinicians can opt for biological alternatives to repair damaged pulps maintaining tissue vitality, sensorial functions, and potential for root development.[12,24,25] Nevertheless, there remain challenges that need to be addressed for the cost-effective clinical translation of tissue engineering strategies for regenerative endodontics.

Immature permanent teeth are obvious candidates for regenerative endodontic procedures. However, preparing the root microenvironment to be beneficial for pulp regeneration, free of infections and undesirable debris, is rather challenging. Although the triple antibiotic paste (1:1:1 ratio of ciprofloxacin, metronidazol, and minocycline) can effectively disinfect the root canal and even to promote revascularization in avulsed teeth, it also presents long-lasting adverse effects on cell survival and proliferation.[60] Similarly, disinfectant solutions such as sodium hypochlorite (NaOCl) may promote the denaturation of proteins and growth factors that are essential for odontoblastic differentiation and pulp regeneration. Moreover, the instrumentation during the chemomechanical preparation may fail to remove microbes invading the dentinal tubules and can make immature teeth more susceptible to fracture.[10,11] However, emerging disinfection strategies may be able create a microbial-free root canal without promoting the denaturation of essential biomolecules and proteins. Such promising scenario has been achieved with the application of nanobubbles with antibacterial nanopolymers or with the use of antibiotic-containing nanofibers in scaffolds for intracanal drug delivery, which can promote significant bacterial death without negatively affecting dental stem cells attachment, proliferation, and apparent regenerative potential.[61,62]

Another aspect that shall be considered is the preparation of the dentin substrate to receive and home cells. The disinfectant solutions can promote the denaturation of biomolecules and proteins present in the dentin matrix. Hence, developing dentin-conditioning protocols to neutralize or reverse the detrimental effects of NaOCl is critical to keep the cell viability and to promote odontoblastic differentiation and tissue regeneration. Moreover, the blood clot formation can be negatively affected by the EDTA irrigation procedure, which can decrease the number and the length of fibrin networks or promote red blood cell deformities.[63] Some of these detrimental effects can be ameliorated by treating the dentin exposed to NaOCl with phosphate-buffered saline followed by an irrigation with 17% EDTA and a final rinse with phosphate-buffered saline. Such protocol has allowed for higher DPSC viability in dentin discs in vitro. The results suggest that the residual effect of EDTA that negatively affects cell viability may be removed by phosphate-buffered saline irrigation.[64] Similar positive effects on blood clot fibrin formation have been observed with a final flushing with saline solution.[63] Hence, further optimization and clinical validation of dentin-conditioning protocols are promising areas for research in regenerative endodontics.

Other area that shall keep evolving is the development of materials and technologies for scaffold preparation. Although inert materials can be used to promote pulp regeneration (**Table 1**,[11,16,30]), the development of bioactive scaffolds able to induce specific biological responses or promote delivery of biomolecules and growth factors can significantly improve cell attachment and migration, odontoblastic differentiation, and dental pulp tissue formation.[18,40,51–53] Notably, it is possible to increase the biological activity of inert polymers such as Polycaprolactone (PCL) by incorporating hydroxyapatite and calcium silicates that are known for their potential to induce odontoblastic differentiation and tissue mineralization (see **Fig. 3**,[52,65,66]). Similarly, the addition of growth factors such as VEGF, TGFβ-1, and BMP-2 in scaffolds can promote endothelial and odontoblastic differentiation, and dentin production.[11,40,67,68] However, mimicking the sequences of events and processes that occur during the formation of a natural dental pulp formation is a daunting challenge. Hence, further research in pulp biology and odontoblastic differentiation are essential to guide the production scaffolds with enhanced biological properties to promote clinically viable strategies for pulp regeneration.

SUMMARY

The development of innovative materials and strategies has led to remarkable achievements in dental pulp tissue engineering. The emergence of new technologies (eg, biochips and bioinks) applied to dental pulp tissue engineering, combined with advancements in scaffold materials and manufacturing techniques, has unveiled new avenues to promote odontoblastic differentiation and the regeneration of functional pulp and dentin in preclinical and clinical studies. Further development in disinfection protocols and bioactive materials and strategies for scaffold production will positively affected the prospects of dental pulp tissue engineering to become a commercially viable clinical alternative.

CLINICS CARE POINTS

- Preclinical and clinical studies have shown that dental pulp tissue engineering strategies have a great potential to become a clinical reality.

- Different strategies (with/without scaffolds or cells) can be used to promote tissue regeneration depending on patient factors (eg, apex shape, age).

- Further developments in material sciences and enabling platforms will keep improving the regenerative potentials and facilitate the clinical adoption of tissue engineering-based strategies for pulp regeneration.

DISCLOSURE

The authors declare no Competing Financial or Non-Financial Interests. This work has been supported by grant from the National University Health System, Singapore (NUHSRO/2020/016/RO5+5/Seed-Aug/14).

REFERENCES

1. Bjorndal L, Simon S, Tomson PL, et al. Management of deep caries and the exposed pulp. Int Endod J 2019;52(7):949–73.
2. Hanna SN, Perez Alfayate R, Prichard J. Vital pulp therapy an insight over the available literature and future expectations. Eur Endod J 2020;5(1):46–53.
3. Medina-Fernandez I, Celiz AD. Acellular biomaterial strategies for endodontic regeneration. Biomater Sci 2019;7(2):506–19.
4. Banchs F, Trope M. Revascularization of immature permanent teeth with apical periodontitis: new treatment protocol? J Endod 2004;30(4):196–200.
5. Orti V, Collart-Dutilleul PY, Piglionico S, et al. Pulp regeneration concepts for non-vital teeth: from tissue engineering to clinical approaches. Tissue Eng B Rev 2018;24(6):419–42.
6. Jeeruphan T, Jantarat J, Yanpiset K, et al. Mahidol study 1: comparison of radio-graphic and survival outcomes of immature teeth treated with either regenerative endodontic or apexification methods: a retrospective study. J Endod 2012; 38(10):1330–6.
7. Altaii M, Richards L, Rossi-Fedele G. Histological assessment of regenerative endodontic treatment in animal studies with different scaffolds: a systematic re-view. Dent Traumatol 2017;33(4):235–44.
8. Saoud TM, Zaazou A, Nabil A, et al. Histological observations of pulpal replace-ment tissue in immature dog teeth after revascularization of infected pulps. Dent Traumatol 2015;31(3):243–9.
9. Kim SG. Biological molecules for the regeneration of the pulp-dentin complex. Dent Clin North Am 2017;61(1):127–41.
10. Galler KM, Buchalla W, Hiller KA, et al. Influence of root canal disinfectants on growth factor release from dentin. J Endod 2015;41(3):363–8.
11. Casagrande L, Demarco FF, Zhang Z, et al. Dentin-derived BMP-2 and odonto-blast differentiation. J Dent Res 2010;89(6):603–8.
12. Xuan K, Li B, Guo H, et al. Deciduous autologous tooth stem cells regenerate dental pulp after implantation into injured teeth. Sci Transl Med 2018;10(455).
13. Chrepa V, Joon R, Austah O, et al. Clinical outcomes of immature teeth treated with regenerative endodontic procedures—a san antonio study. J Endod 2020; 46(8):1074–84.
14. Chan EKM, Desmeules M, Cielecki M, et al. Longitudinal cohort study of regen-erative endodontic treatment for immature necrotic permanent teeth. J Endod 2017;43(3):395–400.
15. Schmalz G, Widbiller M, Galler KM. Clinical perspectives of pulp regeneration. J Endod 2020;46(9S):S161–74.
16. Rosa V, Sriram G, McDonald N, et al. A critical analysis of research methods and biological experimental models to study pulp regeneration. Int Endod J 2022;55: 446–55.
17. Bottino MC, Pankajakshan D, Nor JE. Advanced scaffolds for dental pulp and periodontal regeneration. Dent Clin North Am 2017;61(4):689–711.
18. Soares DG, Bordini EAF, Bronze-Uhle ES, et al. Chitosan-calcium-simvastatin scaffold as an inductive cell-free platform. J Dent Res 2021;100(10):1118–26.

19. Yelick PC, Sharpe PT. Tooth bioengineering and regenerative dentistry. J Dent Res 2019;98(11):1173–82.
20. Itoh Y, Sasaki JI, Hashimoto M, et al. Pulp regeneration by 3-dimensional dental pulp stem cell constructs. J Dent Res 2018;97(10):1137–43.
21. Nakashima M, Iohara K, Bottino MC, et al. Animal models for stem cell-based pulp regeneration: foundation for human clinical applications. Tissue Eng Part B Rev 2019;25(2):100–13.
22. Xie Z, Shen Z, Zhan P, et al. Functional dental pulp regeneration: basic research and clinical translation. Int J Mol Sci 2021;22(16).
23. Botero TM, Nör JE. Tissue engineering strategies for endodontic regeneration. In: Vishwakarma A, Sharpe P, Songtao S, et al, editors. Stem cell biology and tissue engineering in dental sciences. 1st edition. London: Academic Press; 2015. p. 419–30.
24. Rosa V, Botero TM, Nor JE. Regenerative endodontics in light of the stem cell paradigm. Int Dent J 2011;61(Suppl 1):23–8.
25. Rosa V, Della Bona A, Cavalcanti BN, et al. Tissue engineering: from research to dental clinics. Dent Mater 2012;28(4):341–8.
26. Shi S, Robey PG, Gronthos S. Comparison of human dental pulp and bone marrow stromal stem cells by cDNA microarray analysis. Bone 2001;29(6):532–9.
27. Martens W, Wolfs E, Struys T, et al. Expression pattern of basal markers in human dental pulp stem cells and tissue. Cells Tissues Organs 2012;196(6):490–500.
28. Rosa V, Xie H, Dubey N, et al. Graphene oxide-based substrate: physical and surface characterization, cytocompatibility and differentiation potential of dental pulp stem cells. Dent Mater 2016;32(8):1019–25.
29. Madanagopal TT, Tai YK, Lim SH, et al. Pulsed electromagnetic fields synergize with graphene to enhance dental pulp stem cell-derived neurogenesis by selectively targeting TRPC1 channels. Eur Cells Mater 2021;41:216–32.
30. Rosa V, Zhang Z, Grande RH, et al. Dental pulp tissue engineering in full-length human root canals. J Dent Res 2013;92(11):970–5.
31. Dissanayaka WL, Hargreaves KM, Jin L, et al. The interplay of dental pulp stem cells and endothelial cells in an injectable peptide hydrogel on angiogenesis and pulp regeneration in vivo. Tissue Eng A 2015;21(3–4):550–63.
32. Khayat A, Monteiro N, Smith EE, et al. GelMA-Encapsulated hDPSCs and HU-VECs for Dental Pulp Regeneration. J Dent Res 2017;96(2):192–9.
33. Athirasala A, Lins F, Tahayeri A, et al. a novel strategy to engineer pre-vascularized full-length dental pulp-like tissue constructs. Sci Rep 2017;7(1).
34. Bordini EAF, Ferreira JA, Dubey N, et al. Injectable multifunctional drug delivery system for hard tissue regeneration under inflammatory microenvironments. ACS Appl Bio Mater 2021;4(9):6993–7006.
35. Monteiro N, He W, Franca CM, et al. Engineering microvascular networks in LED light-cured cell-laden hydrogels. ACS Biomater Sci Eng 2018;4(7):2563–70.
36. Qu L, Dubey N, Ribeiro JS, et al. Metformin-loaded nanospheres-laden photo-crosslinkable gelatin hydrogel for bone tissue engineering. J Mech Behav Biomed Mater 2021;116:104293.
37. Ribeiro JS, Daghrery A, Dubey N, et al. Hybrid antimicrobial hydrogel as injectable therapeutics for oral infection ablation. Biomacromolecules 2020;21(9):3945–56.
38. Soares DG, Bordini EAF, Swanson WB, et al. Platform technologies for regenerative endodontics from multifunctional biomaterials to tooth-on-a-chip strategies. Clin Oral Investig 2021;25(8):4749–79.

39. Kuang R, Zhang Z, Jin X, et al. Nanofibrous spongy microspheres enhance odontogenic differentiation of human dental pulp stem cells. Adv Healthc Mater 2015; 4(13):1993–2000.

40. Li X, Ma C, Xie X, et al. Pulp regeneration in a full-length human tooth root using a hierarchical nanofibrous microsphere system. Acta Biomater 2016;35:57–67.

41. Zhang Q, Yang T, Zhang R, et al. Platelet lysate functionalized gelatin methacrylate microspheres for improving angiogenesis in endodontic regeneration. Acta Biomater 2021;136:441–55.

42. Abaci A, Guvendiren M. Designing decellularized extracellular matrix-based bioinks for 3D bioprinting. Adv Healthc Mater 2020;9(24):e2000734.

43. Fonseca AC, Melchels FPW, Ferreira MJS, et al. Emulating human tissues and organs: a bioprinting perspective toward personalized medicine. Chem Rev 2020; 120(19):11128–74.

44. Tan Q, Cao Y, Zheng X, et al. BMP4-regulated human dental pulp stromal cells promote pulp-like tissue regeneration in a decellularized dental pulp matrix scaffold. Odontology 2021;109(4):895–903.

45. Bakhtiar H, Rajabi S, Pezeshki-Modaress M, et al. Optimizing methods for bovine dental pulp decellularization. J Endod 2021;47(1):62–8.

46. Matoug-Elwerfelli M, Nazzal H, Raif EM, et al. Ex-vivo recellularisation and stem cell differentiation of a decellularised rat dental pulp matrix. Sci Rep 2020;10(1).

47. Alqahtani Q, Zaky SH, Patil A, et al. Decellularized swine dental pulp tissue for regenerative root canal therapy. J Dent Res 2018;97(13):1460–7.

48. Yuasa K, Fukumoto S, Kamasaki Y, et al. Laminin α2 is essential for odontoblast differentiation regulating dentin sialoprotein expression. J Biol Chem 2004; 279(11):10286–92.

49. Na S, Zhang H, Huang F, et al. Regeneration of dental pulp/dentine complex with a three-dimensional and scaffold-free stem-cell sheet-derived pellet. J Tissue Eng Regen Med 2016;10(3):261–70.

50. Eramo S, Natali A, Pinna R, et al. Dental pulp regeneration via cell homing. Int Endod J 2018;51(4):405–19.

51. Soares DG, Rosseto HL, Scheffel DS, et al. Odontogenic differentiation potential of human dental pulp cells cultured on a calcium-aluminate enriched chitosan-collagen scaffold. Clin Oral Investig 2017;21(9):2827–39.

52. Bhargav A, Min KS, Wen Feng L, et al. Taguchi's methods to optimize the properties and bioactivity of 3D printed polycaprolactone/mineral trioxide aggregate scaffold: theoretical predictions and experimental validation. J Biomed Mater Res B: Appl Biomater 2019;108(3):629–37.

53. Soares DG, Zhang Z, Mohamed F, et al. Simvastatin and nanofibrous poly(l-lactic acid) scaffolds to promote the odontogenic potential of dental pulp cells in an inflammatory environment. Acta Biomater 2018;68:190–203.

54. Widbiller M, Schmalz G. Endodontic regeneration: hard shell, soft core. Odontology 2021;109(2):303–12.

55. Xie H, Dubey N, Shim W, et al. Functional odontoblastic-like cells derived from human iPSCs. J Dent Res 2017;97(1):77–83.

56. Athirasala A, Tahayeri A, Thrivikraman G, et al. A dentin-derived hydrogel bioink for 3D bioprinting of cell laden scaffolds for regenerative dentistry. Biofabrication 2018;10(2):024101.

57. Holiel AA, Mahmoud EM, Abdel-Fattah WM, et al. Histological evaluation of the regenerative potential of a novel treated dentin matrix hydrogel in direct pulp capping. Clin Oral Investig 2021;25(4):2101–12.

58. Syed-Picard FN, Ray HL, Kumta PN, et al. Scaffoldless tissue-engineered dental pulp cell constructs for endodontic therapy. J Dent Res 2014;93(3):250–5.
59. Dissanayaka WL, Zhu L, Hargreaves KM, et al. Scaffold-free prevascularized microtissue spheroids for pulp regeneration. J Dent Res 2014;93(12):1296–303.
60. Ruparel NB, Teixeira FB, Ferraz CC, et al. Direct effect of intracanal medicaments on survival of stem cells of the apical papilla. J Endod 2012;38(10):1372–5.
61. Nakashima M, Iohara K, Zayed M. Pulp regeneration: current approaches, challenges, and novel rejuvenating strategies for an aging population. J Endod 2020; 46(9):S135–42.
62. Pankajakshan D, Albuquerque MTP, Evans JD, et al. Triple antibiotic polymer nanofibers for intracanal drug delivery: effects on dual species biofilm and cell function. J Endod 2016;42(10):1490–5.
63. Taweewattanapaisan P, Jantarat J, Ounjai P, et al. The Effects of EDTA on blood clot in regenerative endodontic procedures. J Endod 2019;45(3):281–6.
64. Aksel H, Albanyan H, Bosaid F, et al. Dentin conditioning protocol for regenerative endodontic procedures. J Endod 2020;46(8):1099–104.
65. Chuenjitkuntaworn B, Inrung W, Damrongsri D, et al. Polycaprolactone/hydroxyapatite composite scaffolds: preparation, characterization, and in vitro and in vivo biological responses of human primary bone cells. J Biomed Mater Res A 2010;94A(1):241–51.
66. Wahl DA, Sachlos E, Liu C, et al. Controlling the processing of collagen-hydroxyapatite scaffolds for bone tissue engineering. J Mater Sci Mater Med 2007;18(2):201–9.
67. Magloire H, Romeas A, Melin M, et al. Molecular regulation of odontoblast activity under dentin injury. Adv Dent Res 2001;15:46–50.
68. Iohara K, Nakashima M, Ito M, et al. Dentin regeneration by dental pulp stem cell therapy with recombinant human bone morphogenetic protein 2. J Dent Res 2004;83(8):590–5.
69. Wu X, Black L, Santacana-Laffitte G, et al. Preparation and assessment of glutaraldehyde-crosslinked collagen–chitosan hydrogels for adipose tissue engineering. J Biomed Mater Res Part A 2007;81A(1):59–65.
70. Lu Q, Pandya M, Rufaihah AJ, et al. Modulation of dental pulp stem cell odontogenesis in a tunable peg-fibrinogen hydrogel system. Stem Cells Int 2015; 2015:1–9.
71. Ehrbar M, Djonov VG, Schnell C, et al. Cell-Demanded Liberation of VEGF from Fibrin implants induces local and controlled blood vessel growth. Circ Res 2004;94(8):1124–32.
72. Jockenhoevel S, Zund G, Hoerstrup SP, et al. Fibrin gel – advantages of a new scaffold in cardiovascular tissue engineering. Eur J Cardiothorac Surg 2001; 19(4):424–30.

Biomaterials for Periodontal Regeneration

Yuejia Deng, BDS, Yongxi Liang, BDS, PhD, Xiaohua Liu, PhD*

KEYWORDS

- Guided bone regeneration • Guided tissue regeneration • Scaffolds • Stem cells
- Collagen barrier • βTCP

KEY POINTS

- Resorbable natural and synthetic barrier membranes have received increasing attractions for use in periodontal regeneration.
- The regeneration of alveolar bone, cementum, and periodontal ligament requires different characteristics of biomaterials.
- More multicentered long clinical studies are needed to provide a better evidence-based clinical guide for biomaterials use.

INTRODUCTION

Periodontitis, which causes the destruction of tooth supporting tissues, is one of the most prevalent chronic diseases in the United States.[1] Patients with periodontitis suffer from the recession of gingival soft tissue, loss of periodontal ligament (PDL), and absorption of alveolar bone. According to the Centers for Disease Control and Prevention, more than 47% of adults aged 30 years and older have some degree of periodontal diseases.[2] Currently, a common procedure for periodontitis treatment is scaling and root planning to remove plaque and calculus above and below the gumline. However, this procedure only delays the progression of local inflammation and cannot recover the lost tooth supporting tissues, including PDL, cementum, and alveolar bone. Therefore, there is an unmet need to reconstruct the damaged/lost periodontal tissues in a clinical setting.

Biomaterial-based approaches have been extensively explored to regenerate periodontal tissues.[3] Guided tissue regeneration/guided bone regeneration (GTR/GBR) has been used for periodontal regeneration for many years.[4] GTR/GBR works by adopting polymeric materials as a physical barrier. This barrier prevents the downgrowth of connective and epithelial tissues into the defective site, therefore favoring the regeneration of periodontal tissues. The effectiveness of the GTR/GBR method

Department of Biomedical Sciences, Texas A&M University College of Dentistry, 3302 Gaston Avenue, Dallas, TX 75246, USA
* Corresponding author.
E-mail address: xliu1@tamu.edu

has been confirmed for vertical alveolar bone loss (3 wall and class II furcation defects)[5] but not for horizontal alveolar bone loss.[6] Meanwhile, current GTR/GBR membranes lack tissue regenerative properties and have to be combined with grafts to enhance tissue regeneration.[4,7,8]

With the advancement of tissue engineering and nanotechnology, new biomimetic materials and scaffolding fabrication technologies that can recapitulate the microenvironment of natural extracellular matrix (ECM) have been developed for periodontal tissue regeneration. This article summarizes recent progress in periodontal regeneration from a biomaterial perspective. First, we provide an overview of GTR/GBR membranes and various natural and synthetic grafting biomaterials that are used for periodontal tissue regeneration. Next, we discuss the recent development of biomaterials and multifunctional scaffolds used for alveolar bone/PDL/cementum regeneration. Finally, we provide clinical care points and perspectives on the use of biomimetic scaffolding materials to reconstruct the hierarchical and functional periodontal tissues.

BIOMATERIALS FOR PERIODONTAL REGENERATION
Barrier Biomaterials

Barrier biomaterials act as a physical barrier to block fast-growing soft tissue cells (epithelial cells and gingival fibroblasts) from growing into defective sites during periodontal regeneration. Besides preventing undesired cell invasion, barrier materials also need to maintain mechanical stability to provide space for periodontal tissue regeneration. GTR/GBR membranes are barrier biomaterials and have been widely used for the treatment of periodontitis. According to the characteristics of degradation, GTR/GBR membranes can be divided into nonresorbable and resorbable barriers. **Table 1** lists the commonly used commercial GTR/GBR membranes.

The first barrier membrane was made from e-PTFE, a material that has excellent biocompatibility and mechanical stability.[9] When high rigidity is required to maintain a large defect space, a titanium framework can be placed between 2 layers of e-PTFE.[10] A recent clinical study adopted a titanium-reinforced microporous e-PTFE (MP-e-PTFE) for vertical ridge augmentation before dental implant placement.[12] Micropores in the e-PTFE were used to reduce bacterial contamination and facilitate removal of the membrane material after tissue regeneration. The results in a 1-year follow-up indicated that the titanium-reinforced MP-e-PTFE membrane is a promising barrier biomaterial for vertical ridge augmentation of severely resorbed ridges within posterior areas.[12] Because PTFE is a non-resorbable membrane, patients need a second surgery to retrieve it, which increases the risk of site morbidity.[20] In addition, e-PTFE membranes have premature exposure rates of 30% to 40%, leading to significant increases in infection, contamination, and impaired bone augmentation.[21] For these reasons, current clinical research is more focused on resorbable membranes.

The most popular resorbable membranes are fabricated from collagen that has high biocompatibility and is capable of promoting wound healing.[11,13–15] Commercial collagen membranes such as Bio-Gide, BioMend, OssGuide, and Genoss have varied collagen types and structures (see **Table 1**). These membranes are resorbed via enzymatic degradation, such as collagenases, macrophage/polymorphonuclear leukocyte-derived enzymes, and bacterial proteases. Collagen membranes promote osteoblastic cell migration and new bone ingrowth.[22] Because collagen is a natural biomaterial, its degradation rate depends on the sources of the material. Generally, collagen membranes have low mechanical strength and a rapid biodegradation rate. Several cross-linking methods have been developed to increase the mechanical properties and decrease the degradation rate.[15,16] The cross-linked collagen

Table 1
A list of the commonly used commercial guided tissue regeneration/guided bone regeneration membranes

Commercial Name	Main Components	Degradation	Application	Reference
Expanded polytetrafluoroethylene (e-PTFE; GORE-TEX®: W.L. Gore & Associates; Flagstaff, AZ,USA)	e-PTFE	Nondegradable	GBR-implant Bone regeneration	Vaibhav et al,[9] 2021
Ti-250(Cytoplast®: Osteogenics Biomedical; Lubbock, USA)	Titanium-reinforced high-density PTFE	Nondegradable	Vertical bone regeneration	Windisch et al,[10] 2021
N-RES (Gore-Tex®: W.L. Gore & Associates; Flagstaff, AZ, USA)	Titanium-reinforced e-PTFE membrane	Nondegradable	GBR	Naenni et al,[11] 2021
TR(OPENTEX® TR: Purgo; Seoul, Korea)	Titanium-reinforced MP-ePTFE	Nondegradable	Vertical Ridge Augmentation	Ji et al,[12] 20201
Bio-Gide®: Geistlich Pharma AG; Wolhusen, Switzerland	Collagen derived from porcine skin	24 wk	Two-wall intrabony defects, GBR	Imber et al,[13] 2021
BioMend®: Zimmer Dental; Carlsbad, CA, USA	Collagen type-I derived from bovine tendon	18 wk	GTR	Foo,[14] 2021
OssGuide®: SK Bioland; Cheonan, Korea	Cross-linked-porcine pericardium-derived type I collagen	12–16 wk	GTR	Lee et al,[15] 2021
Genoss®: Genoss Company Limited; Suwon, Korea	Cross-linked type-I collagen derived from bovine tendon	N/A	GBR-implant Bone regeneration	Cha et al,[16] 2021
Tisseos®: Biomedical Tissues; La Chapelle-sur-Erdre, France	Poly(lactic-co-glycolic acid)	N/A	GBR	Naenn et al,[17] 2020
GUIDOR®: Guidor AB; Huddinge, Sweden	Poly(lactic acid)	6 wk	GBR	Naenni et al,[17] 2020, Di Raimondo et al,[18] 2021
Straumann®: Straumann AG; Basel, Switzerland MembraGel	Polyethylene glycol membrane	N/A	GBR-implant Bone regeneration	Jung et al,[19] 2020

Abbreviations: N-RES, Non-resorbable.

membrane maintained the position of block bone substitutes in the early healing period of an lateral onlay graft.[23] However, research showed that the cross-linked collagen membrane delayed the process of angiogenesis.[24] A recent clinical trial showed that there was no significant difference in ridge preservation when comparing collagen membranes and PTFE.[25]

Other natural resorbable membrane biomaterials that have been tested include gelatin, chitosan, and silk fibroin.[26–28] Gelatin is derived from collagen and has excellent biocompatibility to promote osteoblasts adhesive and growth, make it a promising biomaterial for GTR/GBR.[29] Chitosan is derived from chitin via deacetylation and has high biocompatibility, antimicrobial activity, and wound healing potential.[30] Silk fibroin is a protein extracted from *Bombyx mori* cocoons and possesses excellent biocompatibility as well as oxygen and water vapor permeability.[31] Compared with collagen, these natural biomaterials used as barrier membranes are still at the preclinical stage, and there are no commercial products for GTR/GBR yet.

The major limitations of natural biomaterials are batch-to-batch differences and inferior mechanical properties.[32] To overcome those drawbacks, several synthetic biodegradable polymers have been synthesized for resorbable GTR/GBR membranes. These polymers include poly(lactic acid), poly(glycolic acid), polyethylene glycol membrane, poly(ε-caprolactone) (PCL), poly(lactic-co-glycolic acid) (PLGA), and their copolymers. However, these synthetic biomaterials lack cell recognition cues and often need surface modification to enhance cell–material interactions. Currently, there are a few commercially available synthetic resorbable membranes on market and many more synthetic polymer membranes are under the animal study phase or in preclinical trials.

Membrane-related infection is the main reason for clinical failure of GTR/GBR due to the complicated biofilm environment in the oral cavity. Recent studies have incorporated different bioactive components to the GTR/GBR membranes to acquire sufficient antibacterial properties. A study added magnesium oxide nanoparticles (NPs) into PCL/gelatin membranes using a coaxial electrospinning technique to enhance antibacterial activity.[33] Similarly, ZnO NPs were introduced into chitin as an antibacterial component to form a functional barrier membrane.[34] The ZnO NPs in the barrier membrane displayed a good antibacterial activity by slowly releasing Zn^{2+} and improved osteogenic capability in a rat periodontal defect model.[34] However, the periodontal bone defect was only partially repaired after the ZnO-containing barrier membrane was completely degraded, indicating the necessity of tailoring the degradation rate of the barrier membrane. Surface coating is another approach to incorporate antimicrobial silver NPs into GTR/GBR membranes.[35] The in vitro experiment demonstrated the antimicrobial ability of surface-modified GTR/GBR membrane against *Staphylococcus aureus* and *Escherichia coli*.[35] However, further studies are needed to identify the long-term antibacterial activity in vivo.

Grafting Biomaterials

Graft materials are commonly used with barrier membranes to achieve periodontal regeneration and alveolar ridge reconstruction. The graft materials can be divided into autografts, allografts, xenografts, and alloplastic materials. A comprehensive search shows that there have been 144 bone graft materials for periodontal use in the United States.[36] Among those products, the number of allografts is the highest, followed by alloplastic materials and xenografts. Because autografts are harvested from the own body of the patient, it possesses all the properties required for new tissue regrowth and structural reconstruction and is considered the gold standard. However, second site morbidity and limited quantities of available tissue limits its application. Allografts are harvested from one individual for transplantation to another. Two of the widely used bone allografts are the freeze-dried bone allograft (FDBA) and the demineralized freeze-dried bone allograft (DFDBA). A recent randomized clinical trial shows that corticocancellous FDBA along with a collagen membrane was effective for horizontal augmentation of the edentulous ridge.[37] Furthermore, adding autogenous bone to the FDBA did not significantly increase the quality and quantity of regenerated bone.[37] When used in ridge preservation of nonmolar tooth sites, there was no significant difference in vital bone formation or dimensional changes among cortical FDBA, 50/50 cortical FDBA/cancellous FDBA, and cancellous FDBA.[38] A study that examined the effect of block allografts on the treatment of intrabony defects in periodontitis showed that both the FDBA and DFDBA significantly improved the periodontal prognosis of teeth with intrabony defects at 12 months postsurgery.[39] Another randomized controlled clinical trial compared the healing of nonmolar extraction sites grafted with either FDBA or a 70/30 FDBA/DFDBA in alveolar ridge preservation.[40] The results showed that the 70/30 FDBA/DFDBA had better vital bone formation while providing similar dimensional stability of the alveolar ridge. A long-term evaluation further indicated that the 70/30 FDBA/DFDBA had approximately twice as much vital bone and half as much residual graft material after 18 to 20 weeks of healing compared with only 8 to 10 weeks of healing.[41]

Xenografts are obtained from different species and prepared by various procedures. Two of the most used xenografts in dentistry are deproteinated bovine bone matrix (DBBM) and demineralized porcine bone matrix (DPBM).[42,43] DBBM has been used in GBR and ridge preservation. The combination of DBBM with recombinant human bone morphogenetic protein-2 resulted in similar bone quantity and quality of lateral ridge augmentation when compared with an autogenous bone block.[44] A recent finding suggested that DPBM and DBBM had comparable histomorphometric outcomes and dimensional stability of ridge preservation.[45] A meta-analysis and systematic review concluded that the use of DBBM for site preservation provided no additional benefits in terms of postextraction new bone formation when compared with natural healing.[46] Similar to allografts, the major concerns associated with xenografts are antigenicity and the risk of disease transmission from donor to recipient.

Alloplastic grafts are synthetic materials and can avoid the above disadvantages of allografts and xenografts. In addition, alloplastic grafts are osteoconductive and cost effective. Although there are many graft products that have been approved in the United States,[47] β-tricalcium phosphate (β-TCP), biphasic calcium sulfate (BCS), biphasic calcium phosphate, and hydroxyapatite (HA) are popular alloplastic grafts used in regenerative dentistry. β-TCP is a widely used synthetic bone graft substitute and possesses excellent biocompatibility.[48] β-TCP facilitates the in-growth of cellular and vascular components and has degradation rates similar to the rate of new bone formation.[49,50] A systematic review and meta-analysis found that β-TCP had the potential for additional clinical improvement in probing pocket depth and clinical attachment level compared with open flap debridement in infrabony defects.[51] A multicenter randomized controlled trial compared the efficacy of PLGA-coated β-TCP (PLGA-β-TCP) on alveolar ridge preservation, and the result showed that PLGA-β-TCP had similar outcomes in terms of maintenance of alveolar bone dimensions, feasibility of implant placement, peri-implant bone level stability, and implant survival up to 12 months postloading.[52] A prospective clinical trial on ridge preservation showed that a combination of β-TCP with BCS was superior to natural healing processes in terms of horizontal dimensional changes after 4 months.[53] In addition, a histologic analysis indicated that the percentage of residual graft was relatively small and without evidence of an inflammatory response or graft encapsulation. HA has a chemical

Table 2
Summary of biomaterials used for periodontal tissue regeneration in recent years

Materials	Functions
Au nanoparticles[58]	Regulate inflammatory response and the cross talk between macrophages and PDL cells to inhibit ligature-induced periodontitis
TiO_2[59]	Induce osteogenic differentiation and implant integration
CaF_2[60]	Enhance osteogenic and cementogenic differentiation of PDLSCs
Mg-doped hydroxyapatite[61]	Enhance osteogenesis of PDLSCs
P11–4 peptide[62,63]	Induce PDLSC osteogenic differentiation and periodontal regeneration
Exopolysaccharide[64]	Enhance cell migration and wound healing
Gelatin methacrylate + HA[65]	Induce PDLSCs to differentiate into osteoblasts and promoted new bone formation in nude mice
Chitin + PLGA + nBGC[66]	Regulate degradation and mechanical stability. Enhance osteogenic capacity in bone and cementum layers

Abbreviation: nBGC, nanobioactive glass ceramic; PDLSC, peridontal ligament stem cell.

formula of $Ca_{10}(OH)_2(PO4)_6$ that is almost identical to the inorganic portion of the bone matrix.[54] A clinical and histologic evaluation of the healing of human intrabony defects from a small number of samples indicated that nano-HA had limited potential to promote periodontal regeneration in human intrabony defects.[55] Meanwhile, long-term studies for the efficacy of the calcium phosphate ceramics on periodontal regeneration are currently lacking.

New Biomaterials and Scaffolds for Periodontal Regeneration

As shown above, clinical research of periodontal biomaterials predominantly focuses on applications for alveolar bone regeneration. Currently, most of the studies on the regeneration of cementum/PDL or the whole periodontium is at the preclinical stage.[56] Although conventional biomaterials are still the main sources for periodontal regeneration,[57] there are some new biomaterials that have been developed for cementum/PDL/alveolar bone regeneration in recent years. **Table 2** lists the biomaterials that were recently tested for periodontal tissue regeneration (all are within the last 5 years).

The regeneration of alveolar bone, cementum, and PDL requires biomaterials with different characteristics.[57] Some new biomaterials have been developed for multifunctional purposes. For example, several minerals or metallic compounds were reported to play multifunctional roles in periodontal regeneration, including osteogenesis/cementogenesis enhancement, mineralization regulation, and inflammation regulation.[58–60] Overall, examination of those biomaterials for periodontal application are still at the early stage and some studies even did not have in vivo results.[59–61,64]

Biomaterials need to be fabricated into suitable scaffolds to perform their functions. A scaffold provides a biomimetic microenvironment to guide periodontal tissue repair and regeneration. Obviously, the periodontium has a hierarchical structure that contains both soft and hard tissues, making it complicated to design the scaffold. For example, a scaffold for alveolar bone and PDL regeneration should have one side to promote osteoblast differentiation and mineralization, whereas the other side to promote antimineralization and enhance PDL formation. Considerable progress has been made in scaffolding design for periodontal regeneration during the last decade.

These scaffolds were generally fabricated into multilayered structures.[66] For example, a trilayered scaffold was designed to regenerate both hard (cementum and alveolar bone) and soft (PDL) periodontal tissues (**Fig. 1**). In that study, the chitin-(PLGA)/nano-bioactive glass ceramic (nBGC)/cementum protein 1 was for the cementum layer, the chitin–PLGA/fibroblast growth factor 2 (FGF2) was for the PDL layer, and the chitin–PLGA/nBGC/Platelet-rich plasma (PRP) was for the alveolar bone layer. The trilayered composite scaffold with growth factors showed complete defect closure and the formation of new cementum, fibrous PDL, and alveolar bone after implantation of 3 months in a rabbit periodontal defect model.[66]

Electrospinning is a widely used method in fabricating scaffolds with nanofibrous architecture that mimics the structure of the natural ECM, which has been proved to be beneficial for many biological functions.[67] Its surface-to-volume ratio of the nanofibrous membrane allows more protein absorption and provides more binding sites to cell receptors.[68] One limitation of electrospinning is its difficulty in generating macropores inside the scaffold for alveolar bone regeneration. Therefore, electrospinning needs to be combined with other technologies (eg, 3-dimensional [3D] printing) to fabricate multilayered periodontal scaffolds.

3D printing is a rapid process that allows precise control over the shape and porosity of a scaffold. A biomimetic 3D printing scaffold was developed to regenerate alveolar bone-PDL-cementum complex structure (**Fig. 2**). When the scaffold was combined with human gingival fibroblasts transduced with AdCMV (AdCMV)-Bone

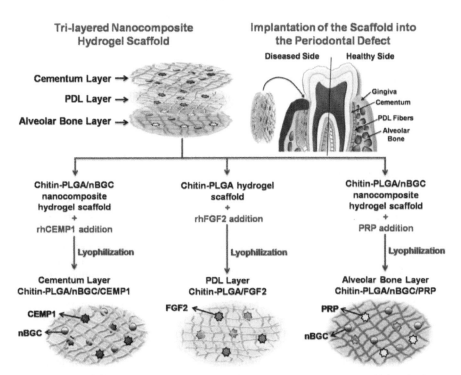

Fig. 1. Design of trilayered membranes to regenerate cementum, PDL, and alveolar bone. (*Adapted from* Sowmya S, Mony U, Jayachandran P, et al. Tri-Layered Nanocomposite Hydrogel Scaffold for the Concurrent Regeneration of Cementum, Periodontal Ligament, and Alveolar Bone. *Adv Healthc Mater.* 2017;6(7).)

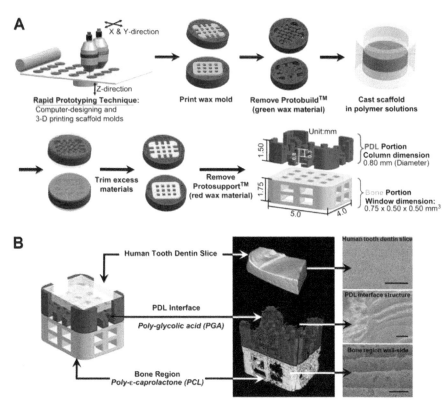

Fig. 2. Three-dimensional printing hybrid scaffolds for periodontal tissue regeneration. (*A*) Schematic illustration of printing hybrid scaffolds. (*B*) Assembly of the hybrid scaffold with a human tooth dentin slice for periodontal tissue regeneration. (*Adapted from* Park CH, Rios HF, Jin Q, et al. Biomimetic hybrid scaffolds for engineering human tooth-ligament interfaces. *Biomaterials.* 2010;31(23):5945-5952.)

morphogenetic protein 7 (BMP7), it formed tooth cementum-like tissue, ligament, and bone structures, indicating the promising of the use of customized periodontal scaffolds for regenerating multitissue interfaces.[69] However, in vivo results showed that the aligned collagen fibers were deposited parallel to the dentin surface. A technology named melt electrowritten (MEW) was recently developed to bridge the gap between solution electrospinning and 3D printing.[70] Because a high voltage is added at the tip of jet, the MEW filaments display a smaller diameter than that of the fibers directly printed from fused-deposition modeling. The MEW enables the deposition of straight polymeric fibers in a layer-by-layer manner and the introduction of well-defined macropores in 3D matrices. However, the MEW is a melt-based additive manufacture process that forms the fibers with diameters at a micrometer level that cannot truly mimic the nanofibrous architecture of ECM. Meanwhile, the compressive yield strength of the polycaprolactone scaffolds fabricated from the MEW was only 1 to 3 kPa,[71] which needs to be significantly increased before the practical application. Overall, the 3D printing and the utilization of a biphasic or triphasic scaffold for periodontal regeneration is still in the early phases of development. More advanced technologies and in vivo studies (especially with the use of a disease model) are necessary to move this research forward in the future.

SUMMARY

Periodontal tissue regeneration requires functional regeneration of tooth supporting periodontium, which contains cementum, connective PDL, and alveolar bone as well as surrounding soft tissues.[72] Biomaterials play a pivotal role in preventing undesired epithelial and gingival fibroblast cell migration as well as guiding other periodontal tissue regeneration. Currently, biomaterials used in clinical settings are mainly focused on physical barrier functions using the GBR/GTR approach. Although nonresorbable membranes are still widely used in clinical practice, resorbable natural and synthetic membranes have become increasingly attractive because they avoid secondary surgery and meet minimally invasive surgery requirements. However, the outcomes of using resorbable barrier membranes varied in different cases according to the defect severity and heterogeneity of patients.[73]

Choosing an ideal grafting material is challenging because each grafting material has advantages and limitations. A suitable bone grafting material should be biocompatible, osteoconductive, osteoinductive, and resorbable.

Multifunctional and multiphasic scaffolds have been designed to regenerate the whole periodontium, including alveolar bone, cementum, and PDL. Mimicking the nanofibrous architecture of natural ECM during scaffolding design provides a better microenvironment for cell proliferation, differentiation, and new tissue formation. Constructing scaffolds with microgrooves and microchannels is a strategy in guiding PDL fiber formation. Temporally and spatially controlled drug/growth factor delivery from multiphasic scaffolds is essential in guiding the growth and differentiation of each cell type in the periodontal defective area. Bioactive NPs are incorporated into the scaffold to enhance the antioxidation, anti-inflammation, antibacterial activities, and angiogenic potential.[74] However, most of the studies related to new biomaterials and scaffolds are in their early phases and more in vivo experiments are needed before clinical trials.

CLINICS CARE POINTS

- Both non-resorbable and resorbable GTR membranes are used in daily practice depending on the need of the case.
- GTR membranes combined with bone grafts enhance tissue regeneration.
- Further in vivo and clinical studies are needed to provide a better evidence-based clinical guide for biomaterial selection.

ACKNOWLEDGMENTS

This study was supported by National Institute of Dental and Craniofacial Research (NIDCR) grant numbers DE024979 and DE029860 (X. Liu). The authors thank Meghann Holt for her assistance with the editing of this article.

DISCLOSURE

No competing financial interests exist.

REFERENCES

1. Eke PI, Dye BA, Wei L, et al. Update on prevalence of periodontitis in adults in the United States: NHANES 2009 to 2012. J Periodontol 2015;86(5):611–22.

2. Kim J, Amar S. Periodontal disease and systemic conditions: a bidirectional relationship. Odontology 2006;94(1):10–21.
3. Chang B, Ahuja N, Ma C, et al. Injectable scaffolds: preparation and application in dental and craniofacial regeneration. Mater Sci Eng R-Reports 2017;111:1–26.
4. Bottino MC, Thomas V, Schmidt G, et al. Recent advances in the development of GTR/GBR membranes for periodontal regeneration-A materials perspective. Dent Mater 2012;28(7):703–21.
5. Sam G, Pillai BR. Evolution of barrier membranes in periodontal regeneration-"Are the third Generation Membranes really here?". J Clin Diagn Res 2014;8(12): Ze14–7.
6. Needleman IG, Worthington HV, Giedrys-Leeper E, et al. Guided tissue regeneration for periodontal infra-bony defects. Cochrane Database Syst Rev 2006;(2): CD001724.
7. Elgali I, Omar O, Dahlin C, et al. Guided bone regeneration: materials and biological mechanisms revisited. Eur J Oral Sci 2017;125(5):315–37.
8. Susin C, Wikesjo UM. Regenerative periodontal therapy: 30 years of lessons learned and unlearned. Periodontol 2000 2013;62(1):232–42.
9. Vaibhav V, Sinha A, Bolisetty D, et al. Osseointegration of dental implants in ridges with insufficient bones using different membranes for guided bone regeneration. J Pharm Bioallied Sci 2021;13(Suppl 1):S225–8.
10. Windisch P, Orban K, Salvi GE, et al. Vertical-guided bone regeneration with a titanium-reinforced d-PTFE membrane utilizing a novel split-thickness flap design: a prospective case series. Clin Oral Investig 2021;25(5):2969–80.
11. Naenni N, Stucki L, Hüsler J, et al. Implants sites with concomitant bone regeneration using a resorbable or non-resorbable membrane result in stable marginal bone levels and similar profilometric outcomes over 5 years. Clin Oral Implants Res 2021;32(8):893–904.
12. Ji JG, Yu JA, Choi SH, et al. Clinical, radiographic, and histomorphometric evaluation of a vertical ridge augmentation procedure using a titanium-reinforced microporous expanded polytetrafluoroethylene membrane: a prospective case series with 1-year follow-up. Materials (Basel) 2021;14(14):3828.
13. Imber JC, Bosshardt DD, Stähli A, et al. Pre-clinical evaluation of the effect of a volume-stable collagen matrix on periodontal regeneration in two-wall intrabony defects. J Clin Periodontol 2021;48(4):560–9.
14. Foo LH. Second attempt of guided tissue regeneration on a previous successfully grafted site with periodontal breakdown-a 5-year follow-up. Eur J Dent 2021; 15(4):806–11.
15. Lee I-K, Choi H-S, Jeong S-H, et al. Evaluating change of marginal bone height with cone-beam computed tomography following surgical treatment with guided tissue regeneration (bone grafting) or access flap alone: a retrospective study. Medicina 2021;57(9):869.
16. Cha JK, Pla R, Vignoletti F, et al. Immunohistochemical characteristics of lateral bone augmentation using different biomaterials around chronic peri-implant dehiscence defects: an experimental in vivo study. Clin Oral Implants Res 2021;32(5):569–80.
17. Naenni N, Lim HC, Strauss FJ, et al. Local tissue effects of various barrier membranes in a rat subcutaneous model. J Periodontal Implant Sci 2020;50(5): 327–39.
18. Di Raimondo R, Sanz-Esporrín J, Sanz-Martin I, et al. Hard and soft tissue changes after guided bone regeneration using two different barrier membranes: an experimental in vivo investigation. Clin Oral Investig 2021;25(4):2213–27.

19. Jung RE, Mihatovic I, Cordaro L, et al. Comparison of a polyethylene glycol membrane and a collagen membrane for the treatment of bone dehiscence defects at bone level implants-A prospective, randomized, controlled, multicenter clinical trial. Clin Oral Implants Res 2020;31(11):1105–15.

20. Rakhmatia YD, Ayukawa Y, Furuhashi A, et al. Current barrier membranes: titanium mesh and other membranes for guided bone regeneration in dental applications. J Prosthodont Res 2013;57(1):3–14.

21. Naung NY, Shehata E, Van Sickels JE. Resorbable versus nonresorbable membranes: when and why? Dent Clin North Am 2019;63(3):419–31.

22. Schlegel AK, Möhler H, Busch F, et al. Preclinical and clinical studies of a collagen membrane (Bio-Gide). Biomaterials 1997;18(7):535–8.

23. Cha JK, Joo MJ, Yoon S, et al. Sequential healing of onlay bone grafts using combining biomaterials with cross-linked collagen in dogs. Clin Oral Implants Res 2017;28(1):76–85.

24. Schwarz F, Rothamel D, Herten M, et al. Angiogenesis pattern of native and cross-linked collagen membranes: an immunohistochemical study in the rat. Clin Oral Implants Res 2006;17(4):403–9.

25. Arbab H, Greenwell H, Hill M, et al. Ridge preservation comparing a nonresorbable PTFE membrane to a resorbable collagen membrane: a clinical and histologic study in humans. Implant Dent 2016;25(1):128–34.

26. Zhang S, Huang Y, Yang X, et al. Gelatin nanofibrous membrane fabricated by electrospinning of aqueous gelatin solution for guided tissue regeneration. J Biomed Mater Res A 2009;90(3):671–9.

27. Qasim SB, Delaine-Smith RM, Fey T, et al. Freeze gelated porous membranes for periodontal tissue regeneration. Acta Biomater 2015;23:317–28.

28. Kim KH, Jeong L, Park HN, et al. Biological efficacy of silk fibroin nanofiber membranes for guided bone regeneration. J Biotechnol 2005;120(3):327–39.

29. Liu X, Smith LA, Hu J, et al. Biomimetic nanofibrous gelatin/apatite composite scaffolds for bone tissue engineering. Biomaterials 2009;30(12):2252–8.

30. Xu C, Lei C, Meng L, et al. Chitosan as a barrier membrane material in periodontal tissue regeneration. J Biomed Mater Res B Appl Biomater 2012;100(5): 1435–43.

31. Jin HJ, Chen J, Karageorgiou V, et al. Human bone marrow stromal cell responses on electrospun silk fibroin mats. Biomaterials 2004;25(6):1039–47.

32. Liu XH, Ma PX. Polymeric scaffolds for bone tissue engineering. Ann Biomed Eng 2004;32(3):477–86.

33. Peng W, Ren S, Zhang Y, et al. MgO nanoparticles-incorporated PCL/gelatin-derived coaxial electrospinning nanocellulose membranes for periodontal tissue regeneration. Front Bioeng Biotechnol 2021;9:668428.

34. Wu T, Huang L, Sun J, et al. Multifunctional chitin-based barrier membrane with antibacterial and osteogenic activities for the treatment of periodontal disease. Carbohydr Polym 2021;269:118276.

35. Nardo T, Chiono V, Carmagnola I, et al. Mussel-inspired antimicrobial coating on PTFE barrier membranes for guided tissue regeneration. Biomed Mater 2021; 16(3):035035.

36. Avila-Ortiz G, Elangovan S, Karimbux N. Bone graft substitutes for periodontal use available in the United States. Clin Adv Periodontics 2013;3:187–90.

37. Hashemipoor M, Asghari N, Mohammadi M, et al. Radiological and histological evaluation of horizontal ridge augmentation using corticocancellous freeze-dried bone allograft with and without autogenous bone: a randomized controlled clinical trial. Clin Implant Dent Relat Res 2020;22(5):582–92.

38. Demetter RS, Calahan BG, Mealey BL. Histologic evaluation of wound healing after ridge preservation with cortical, cancellous, and combined cortico-cancellous freeze-dried bone allograft: a randomized controlled clinical trial. J Periodontol 2017;88(9):860–8.

39. Kothiwale S, Bhimani R, Kaderi M, et al. Comparative study of DFDBA and FDBA block grafts in combination with chorion membrane for the treatment of periodontal intra-bony defects at 12 months post surgery. Cell Tissue Bank 2019. https://doi.org/10.1007/s10561-018-09744-5.

40. Borg TD, Mealey BL. Histologic healing following tooth extraction with ridge preservation using mineralized versus combined mineralized-demineralized freeze-dried bone allograft: a randomized controlled clinical trial. J Periodontol 2015; 86(3):348–55.

41. Nelson AC, Mealey BL. A randomized controlled trial on the impact of healing time on wound healing following ridge preservation using a 70%/30% combination of mineralized and demineralized freeze-dried bone allograft. J Periodontol 2020;91(10):1256–63.

42. Nasr HF, Aichelmann-Reidy ME, Yukna RA. Bone and bone substitutes. Periodontol 2000 1999;19:74–86.

43. Lee JH, Yi GS, Lee JW, et al. Physicochemical characterization of porcine bone-derived grafting material and comparison with bovine xenografts for dental applications. J Periodontal Implant Sci 2017;47(6):388–401.

44. Thoma DS, Payer M, Jakse N, et al. Randomized, controlled clinical two-centre study using xenogeneic block grafts loaded with recombinant human bone morphogenetic protein-2 or autogenous bone blocks for lateral ridge augmentation. J Clin Periodontol 2018;45(2):265–76.

45. Lai VJ, Michalek JE, Liu Q, et al. Ridge preservation following tooth extraction using bovine xenograft compared with porcine xenograft: a randomized controlled clinical trial. J Periodontol 2020;91(3):361–8.

46. Zhao H, Hu J, Zhao L. Histological analysis of socket preservation using DBBM. A systematic review and meta-analysis. J Stomatol Oral Maxillofac Surg 2020; 121(6):729–35.

47. Fukuba S, Okada M, Nohara K, et al. Alloplastic bone substitutes for periodontal and bone regeneration in dentistry: current status and prospects. Materials (Basel) 2021;14(5).

48. Snyder AJ, Levin MP, Cutright DE. Alloplastic implants of tricalcium phosphate ceramic in human periodontal osseous defects. J Periodontol 1984;55(5):273–7.

49. Yip I, Ma L, Mattheos N, et al. Defect healing with various bone substitutes. Clin Oral Implants Res 2015;26(5):606–14.

50. LeGeros RZ. Calcium phosphate-based osteoinductive materials. Chem Rev 2008;108(11):4742–53.

51. Liu CC, Solderer A, Heumann C, et al. Tricalcium phosphate (-containing) biomaterials in the treatment of periodontal infra-bony defects: a systematic review and meta-analysis. J Dent 2021;114:103812.

52. Saito H, Couso-Queiruga E, Shiau HJ, et al. Evaluation of poly lactic-co-glycolic acid-coated β-tricalcium phosphate for alveolar ridge preservation: a multicenter randomized controlled trial. J Periodontol 2021;92(4):524–35.

53. Mayer Y, Zigdon-Giladi H, Machtei EE. Ridge preservation using composite alloplastic materials: a randomized control clinical and histological study in humans. Clin Implant Dent Relat Res 2016;18(6):1163–70.

54. Rajula MPB, Narayanan V, Venkatasubbu GD, et al. Nano-hydroxyapatite: a driving force for bone tissue engineering. J Pharm Bioallied Sci 2021;13(Suppl 1):S11–4.

55. Horváth A, Stavropoulos A, Windisch P, et al. Histological evaluation of human intrabony periodontal defects treated with an unsintered nanocrystalline hydroxyapatite paste. Clin Oral Investig 2013;17(2):423–30.

56. Li Q, Yang G, Li J, et al. Stem cell therapies for periodontal tissue regeneration: a network meta-analysis of preclinical studies. Stem Cel Res Ther 2020;11(1):427.

57. Liang Y, Luan X, Liu X. Recent advances in periodontal regeneration: a biomaterial perspective. Bioact Mater 2020;5(2):297–308.

58. Ni C, Zhou J, Kong N, et al. Gold nanoparticles modulate the crosstalk between macrophages and periodontal ligament cells for periodontitis treatment. Biomaterials 2019;206:115–32.

59. Elango J, Selvaganapathy PR, Lazzari G, et al. Biomimetic collagen-sodium alginate-titanium oxide (TiO2) 3D matrix supports differentiated periodontal ligament fibroblasts growth for periodontal tissue regeneration. Int J Biol Macromol 2020; 163:9–18.

60. Liu J, Dai Q, Weir MD, et al. Biocompatible nanocomposite enhanced osteogenic and cementogenic differentiation of periodontal ligament stem cells in vitro for periodontal regeneration. Materials (Basel) 2020;13(21):495.

61. Shoba E, Lakra R, Kiran MS, et al. 3 D nano bilayered spatially and functionally graded scaffold impregnated bromelain conjugated magnesium doped hydroxyapatite nanoparticle for periodontal regeneration. J Mech Behav Biomed Mater 2020;109:103822.

62. El-Sayed B, Davies RPW, El-Zehery RR, et al. An in-vivo intraoral defect model for assessing the use of P11-4 self-assembling peptide in periodontal regeneration. Front Bioeng Biotechnol 2020;8:559494.

63. Koch F, Meyer N, Valdec S, et al. Development and application of a 3D periodontal in vitro model for the evaluation of fibrillar biomaterials. BMC Oral Health 2020;20(1):148.

64. Kibar H, Arslan YE, Ceylan A, et al. Weissella cibaria EIR/P2-derived exopolysaccharide: a novel alternative to conventional biomaterials targeting periodontal regeneration. Int J Biol Macromol 2020;165(Pt B):2900–8.

65. Chen X, Bai S, Li B, et al. Fabrication of gelatin methacrylate/nanohydroxyapatite microgel arrays for periodontal tissue regeneration. Int J Nanomedicine 2016;11: 4707–18.

66. Sowmya S, Mony U, Jayachandran P, et al. Tri-layered nanocomposite hydrogel scaffold for the concurrent regeneration of cementum, periodontal ligament, and alveolar bone. Adv Healthc Mater 2017;6(7):1601251.

67. Agarwal S, Wendorff J, Greiner A. Use of electrospinning technique for biomedical applications. Polymer 2008;49(26):5603–21.

68. Ekambaram R, Paraman V, Raja L, et al. Design and development of electrospun SPEEK incorporated with aminated zirconia and curcumin nanofibers for periodontal regeneration. J Mech Behav Biomed Mater 2021;123:104796.

69. Park CH, Rios HF, Jin Q, et al. Biomimetic hybrid scaffolds for engineering human tooth-ligament interfaces. Biomaterials 2010;31(23):5945–52.

70. Brown TD, Dalton PD, Hutmacher DW. Direct writing by way of melt electrospinning. Adv Mater 2011;23(47):5651–7.

71. Abbasi N, Abdal-Hay A, Hamlet S, et al. Effects of Gradient and offset architectures on the mechanical and biological properties of 3-D melt electrowritten (MEW) scaffolds. ACS Biomater Sci Eng 2019;5(7):3448–61.

72. Catón J, Bostanci N, Remboutsika E, et al. Future dentistry: cell therapy meets tooth and periodontal repair and regeneration. J Cell Mol Med 2011;15(5): 1054–65.

73. Aprile P, Letourneur D, Simon-Yarza T. Membranes for guided bone regeneration: a road from bench to bedside. Adv Healthc Mater 2020;9(19):e2000707.

74. Fathi-Achachelouei M, Knopf-Marques H, Ribeiro da Silva CE, et al. Use of nano-particles in tissue engineering and regenerative medicine. Front Bioeng Bio-technol 2019;7:113.

Assuring the Safety of Dental Materials

The Usefulness and Application of Standards

Spiro J. Megremis, PhD, MS

KEYWORDS

- ANSI/ADA standards • ISO standards • Dental research • Vertical standards
- Horizontal standards • Technical report • ADA • FDA

KEY POINTS

- Dental material standards have a more than 100-year history in the United States and are informed by scientific research.
- Dental material standards are developed by working groups comprised volunteers from diverse interest groups, including industry, academia, government, and you, the practicing dentist.
- If a company claims that their material passes the American National Standards Institute/American Dental Association or International Organization for Standardization standard, the information provided in their marking, labeling, and instructions for use should allow you to make informed decisions about how to safely and effectively use their products.
- Once you understand how to look up dental product categories through the Food and Drug Administration (FDA) Web site, it is relatively easy to see if your dental material has been cleared by the FDA.
- It is buyer beware when it comes to purchasing dental materials and devices over the Internet.

The formal history of standards and dentistry in the United States goes back to World War I and was prompted by the government's need to buy large quantities of dental materials to treat "an army of teeth in disrepair."[1] This article covers the use of scientific research to establish specifications and standards used to evaluate dental materials and products, and how a practitioner can use these standards to assure the safety and performance of the materials that they use in their everyday practice.

BRIEF HISTORY OF DENTAL RESEARCH AND STANDARDS

The formal amalgamation (pun intended) of scientific research to inform standards development for dental materials began at the National Bureau of Standards (NBS)

Dental Materials & Devices Research, ADA Science & Research Institute (ADA SRI), LLC, 211 East Chicago Avenue, Chicago, IL 60611, USA
E-mail address: megremiss@ada.org

Dent Clin N Am 66 (2022) 673–689
https://doi.org/10.1016/j.cden.2022.05.012
0011-8532/22/© 2022 Elsevier Inc. All rights reserved.

in late 1917 at the request of the Surgeon General of the Army to address "the woeful state of soldiers' teeth."[1,2] Dr Wilmer Souder, a physicist at the NBS, was given the task of leading research to characterize dental amalgam, which eventually led to the first dental specification by the American Dental Association (ADA) on dental amalgam in 1926.[2] After the war, in 1922, Dr Souder and his colleague, Dr Peter Hidnert, expanded NBS scientific research into characterizing the behavior of other dental materials, including inlay materials, plasters, and waxes.[1] By 1928, the ADA officially entered into a collaboration with the NBS, which continues through the present day, and has included the participation of "research associates" from the ADA as well as other government agencies, organizations, and institutions, such as the US Navy, the Air Force, and the National Association of Dental Laboratories.[2] Before this work began, it was reported that the rejection of dental materials tested at the NBS for the US Government was as high as 50% or more.[1] Furthermore, the same book on the history of the NBS states that the Commerce Department suppressed an NBS report that would have revealed that "6 out of 10 dental amalgams available to the profession were unsatisfactory, and only 4 out of 10 would stay in any appreciable time if used as fillings."[1]

However, by the early 1930s, the rejection of amalgam materials amounted to less than 10%, and an NBS Annual Report from that time stated the following[1]:

> [it became] possible for dentists to use amalgam fillings that [would] not shrink and drop out, cements that [would] not dissolve, bridgework that [was] practically permanent, and gold inlays lasting [far beyond the] 3 to 5 years as was the case a short time ago.

This brief history of the work that began at the NBS, which is now the National Institute of Standards and Technology, strikingly demonstrates the importance of the collaboration of dental research and standards to produce "satisfactory" dental materials. Without standards that set minimum requirements to characterize a safe and effective dental material, it is difficult for the practitioner to know what they are getting. The first 50 years of the collaboration between the NBS, ADA, and other stakeholders produced 25 standards addressing dental materials along with more than 600 scientific papers.[2] In 2022, one hundred years after Souder and Hidnert expanded the scientific investigations on dental materials at the NBS that led to the first standard on dental amalgam, the ADA cites well over 100 American National Standards Institute (ANSI)/ADA standards and ADA technical reports (TRs) on dental products.[3] Over that time period, US dental standards development teams have expanded from that small group of NSB and ADA scientists to over 300 volunteers from the profession, industry, academia, and government developing standards through a consensus-based process, as explained in the following section.[4] An important part of the mix is the oral health profession represented by practicing dentists and experts from oral health research, with the latter being the subject of a 2021 editorial in the *Journal of Dental Research* calling for increased involvement "to provide methodological knowledge and experience, balance the interests of other stakeholders, and finally improve oral health."[5] The composition of standards working groups (WGs) and the methods they use to develop standards is discussed in the next section.

HOW STANDARDS ARE DEVELOPED

After the publication of the first dental specification on dental amalgam by the ADA, the progression of US dental standards continued to be directed by the Dental Division of the NBS in collaboration with the ADA.[2,6] Then, in 1953, at the request of the ADA, the

Dental Materials Group (DMG) of the International Association of Dental Research began direct involvement in the development of ADA specifications, also known as vertical standards (defined later), instead of just providing comments during a review period following their drafting.[6] As a result of the ADA request, an arrangement was established between the ADA and the DMG to develop specifications through a committee, with Dr George Paffenbarger, the director of the ADA research unit at the NBS and first professional dentist to engage in research there, as the first Secretary of the committee.[2,6] This position was held by Paffenbarger until 1964, when Dr John Stanford, the Secretary of the ADAs Council on Dental Materials, took over the responsibilities.[6]

In 1962, international involvement in the development of dental standards was increasing with the establishment of the International Organization for Standardization (ISO) Technical Committee (TC) 106 for Dentistry.[7] As a result of this increased international activity, a conference was held in 1969 at ANSI with the purpose of forming a nationally recognized standards body for dentistry in the United States with the formal help and support of ANSI.[6] As a result of this meeting, from 1970 to the present day, the ADA has developed standards through a consensus process using standards committees, and in 2000, the ADA was officially approved as an ANSI-accredited standards developing organization.[6,8] ANSI is the standardization body that is the US member to ISO, and ANSI has the responsibility of accrediting US Technical Advisory Groups (TAGs) to serve as the national mirror committees in relation to ISO TCs.[9,10] ANSI has designated the ADA as sponsor and Secretariat of the US TAG for ISO/TC 106 Dentistry.[9] This gives the United States a voice and vote for the development of international standards for dentistry.

It is interesting that the existence of ANSI approximately coincides with the beginning of Souder's scientific work on dental materials; ANSI was established in 1918 as the American Engineering Standards Committee (AESC) by the American Society for Testing and Materials, along with four other engineering organizations and three federal agencies, including the Department of Commerce, which was in charge of the NSB, where Souder was doing his work.[1,11] Before being renamed ANSI in 1969, AESC became the American Standards Association, and it was under this name that the organization came together with 24 other standards organizations from around the world to form ISO, shortly after the end of World War II.[11] The purpose of ANSI is to serve as an impartial national body to coordinate standards development and approve national consensus standards.[11] The ADA is one of approximately 240 ANSI-accredited standards developers that develop American National Standards in accordance with ANSIs Essential Requirements, which include stipulations for consensus, openness, due process, balance, and a lack of dominance, as described below.[12]

Currently, US national standards and TRs that address dental products are developed through the ADA Standards Committee on Dental Products (SCDPs), which has a Scope that includes "Nomenclature, standards, and specifications for dental materials, except those recognized as drugs or dental radiographic film."[4] The SCDP is composedd of nine subcommittees (SCs), as shown in **Box 1**. Each SC is, in turn, composed of individual WGs with the ADA SCDP currently having over 60 WGs.[4] Some popular, active dental materials WGs are polymer-based restorative materials (PBRMs) and dental ceramics within SC1 on restorative and orthodontic materials and SC2 on prosthodontic materials, respectively. Each WG is composed of volunteers from the profession, industry, academia, and government. Practicing dentists can also join a WG and participate in standards development by contacting the ADA Center for Informatics and Standards (ada.org/dentalstandards). WG volunteers are divided into three interest groups defined as follows[9]:

> **Box 1**
> **The nine different subcommittees (SC) that comprise the American Dental Association Standards Committee on Dental Products (ADA SCDP)**
>
> *American Dental Association Standards Committee on Dental Products*
>
> SC1 Restorative and Orthodontic Materials
>
> SC2 Prosthodontic Materials
>
> SC3 Dental Terminology
>
> SC4 Instruments
>
> SC5 Infection Control, Barrier and Safety Products
>
> SC6 Equipment
>
> SC7 Abrasives and Oral Hygiene Devices
>
> SC8 Dental Implants
>
> SC9 CAD/CAM in Dentistry

1. *Producer/industry*: A member who represents an organization that produces or sells materials, products, systems, or services covered in the scope(s) of the document(s) developed within the SC shall be classified as a producer.
2. *Consumer*: A member, or a member who represents an organization, who in the context of his/her profession purchases or uses materials, products, systems, or services covered in the scope(s) of the document(s) developed within the SC shall be classified as a consumer provided that the member could not also be classified as a producer.
3. *General interest*: A member who does not fit into any of the preceding categories, for example, government agency representative, representative of consumer groups, or research experts.

Within these WGs, standards are developed as ANSI/ADA standards according to a consensus body voting with fair and equitable representation by the different interest groups without "dominance" by any single interest group.[9,13] In this case, an absence of dominance is demonstrated by a "reasonable balance" of participation by the different interest groups, without any single interest group demonstrating a position of overriding authority, leadership, and influence through exercising superior leverage, strength, or representation.[9] Furthermore, a reasonable balance is assumed, with no test for dominance being necessary unless there is a claim made of single interest dominance by a directly and materially affected person.[9]

Historically, once the ADA and the DMG began developing dental materials standards within a specifications committee, the procedure for developing an individual standard for a class of materials was to test existing materials that were performing satisfactorily in the dental market at the time.[14,15] The range of values obtained from performing various tests to characterize these existing materials would then be used as requirements in the standard along with the test methods themselves and composition requirements.[15] Technically, at the time, these documents were called specifications, although they were essentially what are now termed as vertical standards.[14] The ADA SCDP defines a vertical standard as one "where composition or some other design factor is included,"[14] and it applies to only one particular class of material, such as amalgam.[16] For most of their history, dental materials standards were developed as vertical standards.[15] In the process, a revision of an original specification was only undertaken based on materials available in the marketplace and on the acceptance of significant new research or test methods, as shown in the example in the following paragraph.[15] Furthermore, it was a directive of the early specifications committee that "new clinically successful materials" that did not meet the existing requirements of the specification would necessitate the document's revision or an entirely new specification, which is also shown in the example.[15]

A good example of a vertical standard, or specification, and its progression over the years to other forms of standards is ADA Specification No. 5 for "Dental Casting Gold Alloy." In this specification, the gold casting alloys were classified into four types by their hardness and gold content, with a minimum requirement for gold and metals of the platinum group ranging from 75 wt% for the extra hard alloys (Type IV) to 83 wt% for the soft alloys (Type I).[15,17] The 75 wt% minimum requirement for gold and the other noble metals was based on the belief at the time that to attain acceptable corrosion and tarnish resistance in the oral cavity, it was necessary for a dental casting alloy to be composed of at least this minimum percentage.[18,19] In an early form of this specification, a nonstandard Brinell hardness test was used for the hardness test method.[15] However, by a 1965 adoption of the ADA specification (before the ANSI certification process), Vickers hardness testing was being required in the document.[17] In 1989, a major revision of this specification dropped the compositional requirements along with the word "gold" from the title, and it added a tarnish test and suggested a corrosion test.[18,19] These changes allowed for the possibility of a dental casting alloy with less than 75 wt% of gold and other noble metals to meet the requirements of the specification. The Foreword of the revised specification states that "lower cost alternatives have been demanded by dentistry."[20] It then goes on to state that through greater knowledge of raw materials and advances in metallurgy, as well as knowledge of the effects of oral tarnish/corrosion on these materials, a number of alloys and alloy systems have been furnished to the market that "have proven to be viable substitutes for the high gold alloys."[20] In addition to a tarnish test and evaluation of the effect of corrosion on mechanical behavior, there were also requirements added for modulus of elasticity and for inclusion of processing information in the instructions for use (IFU), along with a test for castability.[20] Furthermore, in 1988, the specification went through another revision, which added a requirement for a static immersion corrosion test method along with other smaller changes.[21]

Therefore, over an approximately 40-year time span, Specification No. 5 evolved from a vertical standard based primarily on the composition of one class of material (gold casting alloy) and material behavior requirements to a standard based mostly on material behavior and design factors, such as castability, with the requirements changing over the years to accommodate the demands and reality of the market. The later version of the specification is an example of what the ADA SCDP defines as a semi-horizontal standard, which is a "standard where only a specific class of products is included," and there are no specific composition requirements.[14] Therefore, Specification No. 5 went from being based on a single class of materials, gold casting alloy, to a specific class of products, which is casting alloys for crown and bridgework, including removable partial dentures. Ultimately, the content of Specification No. 5 was incorporated into the horizontal standard ANSI/ADA Standard No. 134 for "Metallic Materials for Fixed and Removable Restorations and Appliances," which covered the content from three former ANSI/ADA specifications with one standard, as described next.[22]

With the creation of the European Union and its standards organization, the European Committee for Standardization (CEN), there was an agreement by CEN to accept standards developed by ISO/TC 106 Dentistry.[14] However, CEN requested ISO/TC 106 consider moving from standards based on classes of materials, or vertical standards, to standards based more on applications, such as horizontal or semi-horizontal standards.[14] In response, in 2000, the ADA SCDP created an *ad hoc* group with the purpose of studying the consequences of changing from vertical to horizontal standards, resulting in a published TR.[14] In this report, they define a horizontal standard as a "standard directed to the application or use," as opposed to one based on a material or class of material, vertical standard, or one based on a specific class of products.[14]

Subsequently, ISO/TC 106, with the cooperation of the US TAG, CEN, and other national standards groups, has been working on developing horizontal standards. A prime example of this is ISO 22674 "*Dentistry–Metallic materials for fixed and removable restorations and appliances*," which was first published in 2006.[23] This document was developed by a WG within *SC2 Prosthodontic materials*, with the active participation of the US TAG. The Foreword states that it replaces the following five composition-derived International Standards[23]: ISO 1562 "Dentistry—Casting gold alloys," ISO 6871-1 "Dental base metal casting alloys—Part 1: Cobalt-based alloys," ISO 6871-2 "Dental base metal casting alloys—Part 2: Nickel-base alloys," ISO 8891 "Dental casting alloys with noble metal content of at least 25% but less than 75%," and ISO 16744 "Dentistry—Base materials for fixed dental restorations." The scope of ISO 22674 covers metallic materials that are suitable for the fabrication of dental appliances and restorations, including ones recommended for use with a ceramic veneer, and specifies their classification and requirements, along with requirements concerning packaging, marking, and IFU.[23] Furthermore, the draft of the third edition of the standard states that it applies to products that were produced using additive and subtractive manufacturing.[24] Analogous work was also undertaken in both the PBRM and dental ceramic WGs resulting in similar types of horizontal standards. Example of the Use of Standards to Properly Cure Your Polymer-Based Restorative Material in a following section.

It is noteworthy that after the publication of the TR concerning the consequences of changing from vertical to horizontal standards, a follow-up *ad hoc* group was formed in 2005 with a stated task of advising the SCDP WGs on how to convert from materials standards to performance standards.[15] The TR that was published from this *ad hoc* group generally defined a performance standard as "a listing of the properties required and minimum requirements to assure safety and efficacy in the application."[15] The roadmap they produced provided a functional analysis example with eight major steps to convert from a materials standard to a performance standard.[15] As of yet, there are no ANSI/ADA or ISO/TC 106 standards that are strictly performance standards. An example would be if a standard strictly defined the performance requirements of an inlay restoration, and then any material, regardless of whether it was a metallic material, dental ceramic, or PBRM, could meet it.

Ultimately, it is the recognition of a standard by a regulatory agency for approval of a product that makes the standard important. In the case of dental devices in the United States, it is the Food and Drug Administration (FDA) that recognizes and uses dental standards for the approval of dental products, as presented in the section on FDA Recognized Standards.

THE DIFFERENCE BETWEEN AMERICAN NATIONAL STANDARDS INSTITUTE/ AMERICAN DENTAL ASSOCIATION AND INTERNATIONAL ORGANIZATION FOR STANDARDIZATION DENTAL STANDARDS

With the ability to easily go online and order a dental product from practically anywhere in the world, it is worth clarifying what differences there are between standards developed in the United States through the ADA SCDP and approved as ANSI/ADA standards and ISO dental standards. A 2022 editorial entitled "Caveat emptor when purchasing dental products online" in the *Journal of the American Dental Association* (JADA) warns that "controlling the sale of medical devices purchased online from an overseas marketplace is problematic because purchases are shipped directly to customers," so ultimately it is buyer beware.[25] The subject of FDA "cleared" and "approved" devices is discussed in a later section of this article. However, for a dentist checking to see if a material complies with a national or international standard and which applies when buying a dental material, the simple answer is that at this point there is no practical difference between an ANSI/ADA and ISO Dental Standard most of the time, with some notable exceptions, as explained below.

As detailed in the previous section, it can be seen that dental standards development in the United States has progressed from the very first national dental standard developed at the NBS to active participation in ISO/TC 106 Dentistry through ADA sponsorship of the US TAG for the development of international dental standards. As such, the ADA coordinates the formulation of the US vote on all international dental standards developed in ISO/TC 106.[9] Each vote is then submitted to ANSI, as the official member of ISO.[9] The history of ISO dental standards was briefly introduced above. In addition, the first international dental standard documents were developed through the International Dental Federation (FDI) in the 1950s.[7,16] They produced the first nine such international documents related to the standardization of dental materials.[7,16] Then, in 1962, the ISO formed TC 106 for Dentistry, with a mandate to continue the work of FDI, and now international standards for dentistry are developed through the consensus process in SCs in ISO/TC 106 Dentistry.[7,16] ISO is a nongovernmental organization that is composed of the single most representative standardization body from each participating country, which for ISO/TC 106 is currently 46 countries (31 participating members and 15 observing members).[9,26]

At this point, the majority of the work on the development of standards takes place at the ISO level, with active US participation through the US TAG, using parallel SCs to the ones listed in **Box 1**. The ISO standards are then adopted as ANSI/ADA standards with adoptions being either identical adoptions (typical) or modified adoptions. If the modifications to the ISO standard are significant, the ADA SCDP usually contacts the FDA and urges them to recognize the ANSI/ADA standard over the ISO standard for their Recognized Consensus Standards database (see FDA section below). An example of an identical adoption is ANSI/ADA Standard No. 134, which is identical to ISO 22674.[27,28] Furthermore, as mentioned previously, when this standard was first adopted, it then covered the content of ANSI/ADA Specification No. 5 and ANSI/ADA Specification No. 14 for *"Dental Base Metal Casting Alloy"*, which were then withdrawn, along with the requirements for the performance of metals and alloys used for the metallic component of a metal-ceramic restoration in what was previously ANSI/ADA Standard No. 38 "Metal–Ceramic Systems".[22]

A practical example of the later situation of a modified adoption being preferred for the US national standard occurred during voting for a revision of ANSI/ADA Standard No. 27, which covers PBRMs. In 2005, there was an ADA SCDP WG vote for an identical adoption of the 2000 version of ISO 4049 "Dentistry–PBRMs."[29] The consideration for adoption failed due to negative votes concerning the requirement for radio-opacity. In the version of ANSI/ADA No. 27 that existed at the time, the radio-opacity requirement stated the following[30]:

"If the manufacturer claims that the material is radio-opaque..., the radio-opacity... shall be equal to 2 or more mm thickness of aluminum."

However, a direct adoption of ISO 4049 would reduce this requirement to 1 mm of aluminum. The WG members could not agree on how to deal with the discrepancy between the two documents. Through numerous ADA member dentist calls to the Scientific Information department, ADA researchers that were members of the WG argued that they had anecdotal information that this difference was causing confusion with member dentists. This was especially the case for international companies that were selling PBRMs labeled as "radio-opaque" that were meeting the 1 mm of aluminum requirement instead of 2 mm. Therefore, for many years, there was a difference in terms of a radio-opacity for the national and international standards. Finally, in 2016, a modified adoption of the ISO standard was adopted for ANSI/ADA Standard No. 27, which required that manufacturers claiming radio-opacity must explain the meaning of the term in the manufacturers' IFU (that is, "…1 mm of material having a radio-opacity equivalent to 1 mm of aluminum has a radio-opacity equivalent to that of dentin").[31]

In a 2019 revision of the ISO standard, the packaging requirements were changed to include the explanation above for radio-opacity in the IFU with a further statement that "…2 mm of aluminum is equivalent to enamel."[32] Since this revision, the ADA SCDP WG agreed to adopt the ISO Standard as an identical adoption, resulting in both the US and international standards on PBRMs finally being harmonized.[32,33] Note that one of the minor differences between ANSI/ADA and ISO dental standards is that the latter uses the "Queen's English," or correct English speech, and the former uses American English. For example, the word "radio-opaque" appears as "radiopaque" generally in American English. However, in this case, to avoid confusion in international labeling, both standards use the term "radio-opaque."[32,33]

This example stresses the importance of labeling and referencing the manufacturer's IFU with materials claiming to meet that appropriate material standard. Every PBRM that claims to be radio-opaque and meets the requirements of the ANSI/ADA or ISO standard must include instructions stating the meaning of the term "radio-opaque." The importance of looking at the instructions for ANSI/ADA and ISO-approved dental materials is stressed further in a later example.

WHO PAYS FOR DENTAL STANDARDS?

As a brief aside, it is important to acknowledge how dental standards development is funded. This has been an issue from the beginning of Souder's work on amalgam that led to the first ADA specification. According to a biography of Souder published in *Dental Materials*, when he first approached the ADA about stationing research associates at the NBS in the early 1920s, he was told that the ADA "had no money for such work."[34] However, Souder was able to find a consultant laboratory, Weinstein Research Laboratories, to support a research associate and collaborate on continued work on dental materials.[34] According to his biography, the publication and presentation of this work "created such a sensation" that the ADA finally agreed to fund a research associate to be stationed at the NBS in 1928.[34]

As detailed above, over the next 50 years, the ongoing collaboration between the NBS and the ADA, along with participation from other government agencies, organizations, and institutions, produced 25 standards and more than 600 scientific papers addressing dental materials.[2] Funding was provided by the ADA Foundation, the NBS, and outside agencies, such as the National Institutes of Health.[2] Currently, although the standards development process is a collaborative consensus-based endeavor, the majority of funding for the administration of dental standards as well as laboratory research to inform it comes from dentists who are members of the ADA in the form of membership dues. As ADA membership has decreased over the years and budgets have become tighter, the use of member dues to fund dental standards development continues to be debated.

FOOD AND DRUG ADMINISTRATION RECOGNIZED STANDARDS, SEARCHING FOR FOOD AND DRUG ADMINISTRATION "APPROVED" DENTAL PRODUCTS, AND REPORTING ADVERSE EVENTS

The Food and Drug Modernization Act of 1997 amended the Food, Drug, and Cosmetic Act to allow the FDA to recognize and use consensus standards in its review process of medical devices.[35] In Title 21 of the Code of Federal Regulations (CFR), Chapter 1 on the FDA has a Subchapter H on Medical Devices that classifies dental devices as medical devices under Part 872, which then lists appropriate dental materials.[36] Therefore, generally speaking, dental materials are regulated as medical devices of different classes that are stratified by risk. The FDA guidance document on the "Appropriate Use of Voluntary Consensus Standards in Premarket Submissions for Medical Devices" documents the advantages of the use of consensus standards, including, among other things, "a consensus approach to certain aspects of the evaluation of device safety and effectiveness."[37]

The FDA has a "Recognized Consensus Standards" Web site page linking to a database that can be searched for a list of national and international voluntary consensus standards to which the FDA will accept a Declaration of Conformity (DOC), as shown in **Fig. 1**.[38] The DOC attests that a device conforms to a cited FDA-recognized standard in the following manner[39]: all normative requirements of the standard are met; all testing has been performed; and testing is conducted on a finished device or final finished device. Generally, the use of a DOC with a recognized standard reduces the required documentation in a submission and improves device review.[39]

Also, of greater value to the practicing dentist, the FDA has a database that can be searched for "approved" or "cleared" devices. As previously noted, dental devices are classified as medical devices by the FDA in 21 CFR 872.[36] It is important to understand that the burden is on dentists to assure that the dental devices they purchase, including dental materials, are legally marketed. One way to find out if a dental product has been "cleared" by the FDA for commercial distribution is to go to the FDA database for 510(k) Premarket Notification clearances, as shown in **Fig. 2**.[40] This database provides a listing of all devices the FDA has cleared since the passage of the Medical Device Amendments to the Food, Drug, and Cosmetic in 1976, which was "intended to provide reasonable assurance of the safety and effectiveness of medical devices"[41] (note that devices on the market before May 28, 1976 are "grandfathered," and do not require FDA clearance). For each device type, the FDA has assigned a "Product Code." An efficient way to search the database is to first find the "Product Code" for the dental product that you are looking for by clicking on the highlighted "Product Code" link and going to the "Product Classification" site. Once on this site, the term "Dental" can be entered under "Review Panel" and a search performed that will bring up a few hundred codes, which can be sorted alphabetically. For instance, a dental materials product code of interest is "EIH", which stands for "Powder, Porcelain." This can then be entered as the Product Code in the original database. That is, when on the 510(k) Premarket Notification clearances site,[40] entering the term "Dental" under "Review Panel" to find the Product Code, then, entering "EIH" in "Product Code" and clicking on the "Search" button, yields a complete list of almost 500 cleared dental ceramic products, including glass ceramics, dental zirconia, and porcelains, which can be sorted by "Device Name", "Applicant", "510(k) Number", and "Decision Date."

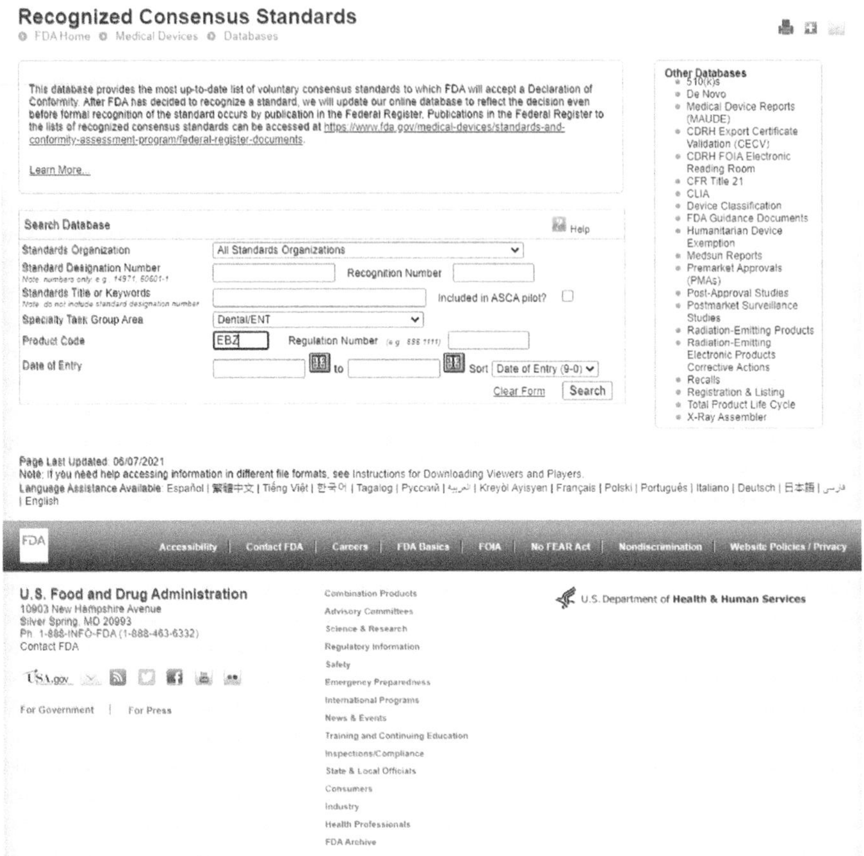

Fig. 1. The FDA Recognized Consensus Standards Database[38] (https://www.accessdata.fda.gov/scripts/cdrh/cfdocs/cfstandards/search.cfm). When on this site, entering "Dental/Ear, Nose, and Throat (ENT)" in the "Specialty Task Group Area" and hitting the "Search" function will return a list of FDA Recognized Consensus Standards for Dental and ENT. This list can then be sorted by "Date of Entry," "Specialty Task Group Area," and "Recognition Number." The standards are then listed by "Standards Developing Organization," "Standard Designation Number and Date," and "Title of Standard." The figure also shows the "Product Code" filled in with "EBZ," which is the code for dental curing units (ultraviolet activator for polymerization). Searching with "Dental/ENT" and "EBZ" entered into the database will return a list of FDA Recognized Consensus Standards for dental curing units.

If you suspect that a dental device, such as one of the dental ceramic materials in the example, has not been cleared by the FDA and is being illegally marketed, you should contact the FDAs Division of Premarket and Labeling Compliance in the Center for Devices and Radiological Health at 301-796-5770, or report it online on the "Report Unlawful Sales of Medical Products on the Internet" webpage.[42] One indicator you can use to determine if a dental device is not legally marketed is to examine the labeling and IFU. If items are missing, poorly written, or if exaggerated claims are made, it is more than likely that the FDA has not cleared the device, as the FDA looks very closely at labeling and IFU as part of their review process (M. Adjodha., Dental Devices Branch of CDRH of the FDA, personal communication, August 17, 2015). Furthermore,

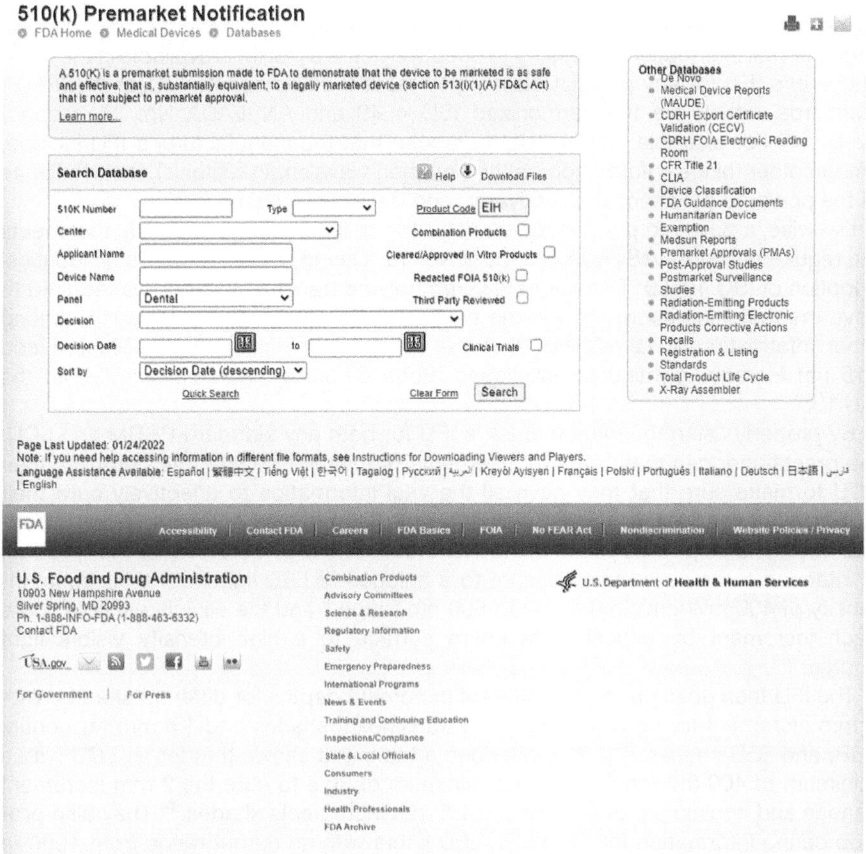

510(k) Premarket Notification

Fig. 2. The FDA database for 510(k) premarket notification[40] (https://www.accessdata.fda.gov/scripts/cdrh/cfdocs/cfPMN/pmn.cfm). This Web site can be used in a couple of practical manners. First, it can be used to search a database for the "Product Code" of dental products, as described in the text. Second, once the specific "Product Code" is known, it can be used on this page to do a specific search. For instance, the Figure shows the "Product Code" populated with "EIH" and "Panel" with "Dental." With these fields filled in, hitting the "Search" button yields a complete list of almost 500 cleared dental ceramic products, including glass ceramics, dental zirconia, and porcelains, which can be sorted by "Device Name," "Applicant," "510(k) Number," and "Decision Date."

if any adverse events occur when using a dental device, you should report this to the FDA through MedWatch, the FDAs gateway for clinically important safety information and for safety alerts, and product recalls.[43] The importance of labeling and IFU will be emphasized in an example in the next section.

EXAMPLE OF THE USE OF STANDARDS TO PROPERLY CURE YOUR POLYMER-BASED RESTORATIVE MATERIAL

There is no universal exposure time for curing all PBRMs.[44] A light-cured PBRM will function as the manufacturer intends only when it receives the required amount of energy at the proper wavelength (that is, the wavelength of the photoinitiator).[45,46]

Additionally, the required amount of light energy to successfully cure a specific PBRM further depends on the formulation, shade, and opacity of the material.[45,46] With that said, the vital information necessary to effectively cure a PBRM is available in the manufacturer's IFU for any product claiming to meet the appropriate ISO or ANSI/ADA standards, which are the harmonized ISO 4049 and ANSI/ADA No. 27, respectively.[32,33] For example, the standards require that the manufacturer's IFU include, among other things, information on the emission wavelength region(s), the irradiance of the powered polymerization activator, and the exposure time.[32,33]

Likewise, a powered polymerization activator, or light-curing unit (LCU), that meets the requirements of ANSI/ADA Standard No. 48 "Curing Lights," which is an identical adoption of ISO 10650 "Dentistry–Powered polymerization activators," is required to have the matching information in the manufacturer's IFU.[47,48] For instance, among other information, it is required that the radiant exitance between 380 nm and 515 nm for each continuous irradiation mode or pulse mode be supplied in the IFU.[47,48]

By properly using the manufacturer's IFU for both any standard PBRM and LCU, the practitioner can match the requirements of their PBRM with the output of their LCU to make sure that they have all the vital information to effectively cure their PBRM. For example, 3M ESPE Filtek Supreme Ultra Universal Restorative is a popular internationally sold PBRM. In the manufacturer's IFU, it states that the "product is intended to be cured by exposure to a halogen or LED light with a minimum intensity of 400 mW/cm^2 in the 400 to 500 nm range," and the clinician should "cure each increment by exposing its entire surface to a high-intensity visible light source."[49]

The IFU then goes on to give different increment depths for different shades, with 2 mm increment for body, enamel, and translucent shades and 1.5 mm for dentin, A6B, and B5B shades.[49] It then provides a table that shows that for an LCU with a minimum of 400 mW/cm^2, it takes a minimum of 20 s to cure the 2 mm increment shades and a minimum of 40 s for the 1.5 mm increments shades.[49] They also provide curing information for 3M ESPE LED lights with an output range from 1000 to 2000 mW/cm^2.[49] Those requirements are a minimum of 10 s to cure the 2 mm increment shades and a minimum of 20 s for the 1.5 mm increments shades.[49] However, as the IFU provides a spectrum of 400 to 500 nm for the required spectral distribution of a compatible curing unit, along with curing times for LCUs with minimum radiant exitance values of 400 mW/cm^2 and 1000 mW/cm^2, then alternative standard LCUs can be used with values listed in their respective IFUs that meet these requirements.

Likewise, Heliomolar by Ivoclar, another common PBRM that exhibits the Conformité Eurōpëenne (CE) mark on its IFU (meaning it meets the requirements of ISO 4049) states that the material should be cured in 2 mm increments with light in the wavelength range of 400 to 500 nm.[50] It then provides a general table with exposure times of 40 and 20 s for LCUs with radiant exitance values of ≥500 mW/cm^2 and ≥1000 mW/cm^2, respectively.[50] Again, this is enough information to know that the Kerr LCU can cure a 2 mm increment in 20 s. This has actually been confirmed by research performed at the ADA laboratories.[45,46] Using a Demi Ultra curing unit, Heliomolar HB (A2 shade) was cured with the LCU centered 2 mm above its surface.[45,46] Using Fourier transform infrared analysis, the average depth of cure was determined to be 2.0 mm.[45,46] The IFU for the Heliomolar product also gives specific curing times for Ivoclar Bluephase LCUs (Style M8, Style, and 20i), which can be verified by matching the information provided in their respective IFUs, as the LCUs also meet the requirements of ISO 10650.[47]

These are just a couple of examples using specific products. However, the important point is that any brands of PBRM and LCU can be substituted into the examples, as long as they meet the appropriate standard. Ultimately, when properly using the IFUs for products that have met the standard, you know that the companies have provided data to a regulatory agency, such as the FDA, that demonstrates that the product performs as intended and is safe. Furthermore, without the knowledge that the material that you are using meets a national or international standard for safety and effectiveness, which has been verified by some regulatory agency, it truly is buyer beware.

IMPORTANT TAKE-HOME POINTS

Dental material standards have a more than 100-year history in the United States and are informed by scientific research. They are developed by WGs composed of volunteers from diverse interest groups, including the industry, academia, government, and you, the practicing dentist.

If a company claims that their material passes the ANSI/ADA or ISO standard, the information provided in their marking, labeling, and IFU should allow you to make informed decisions about how to safely and effectively use their products. And, importantly, when contacted, they should be able to produce any of the information required from the standard that might be missing or is incomplete. In the examples provided on how to use standards to properly cure your PBRM, it can be seen that a curing unit from one company can be used to effectively cure a material from another company, as long as long as the respective products meet the appropriate ANSI/ADA or ISO standards, which both include the vital information in the manufacturer's IFU.

Once you understand how to look up dental product categories through the FDA Web site, it is relatively easy to see if your dental material has been cleared by the FDA. If after searching the FDA Web site you still are not sure about the status of the dental material, you should contact the manufacturer. They should be able to provide proof of their 510(k) clearance. It is buyer beware when it comes to purchasing dental materials and devices over the Internet.

CLINICS CARE POINTS

> - Make sure that the dental materials you use meet the requirements specified in the appropriate ANSI/ADA or ISO standard.
> - If the dental material you are using states that it meets the requirements of the appropriate dental standard, closely follow the manufacturer's IFU to ensure the effectiveness of the product.
> - Since the burden is on the dentist to ensure that the dental device they purchase, including dental materials, is legally marketed, search the FDA database to see if the dental material you intend on purchasing has been cleared by the FDA, as shown in this article.
> - Since dental standards have specific labeling and IFU requirements and the FDA looks very closely at labeling and IFU as part of their review process, it is unlikely that the FDA has cleared any product for which items are missing, poorly written, or exaggerated claims are made.
> - Dental standards allow different dental products to be used effectively together. In this article, it is shown that dental standards allow a curing unit from one company to effectively cure a PBRM from another company, as long as the respective products meet the appropriate dental standards and you closely follow the approved manufacturers' IFUs.

ACKNOWLEDGMENTS

Dr Terry Woods, Chief Engineer for Standards and Strategic Outreach, FDA Center for Devices and Radiological Health for review of FDA content. Sharon Stanford, Director, Standards, Center for Informatics and Standards, ADA and Kathy Medic, Manager, Dental Materials Standards, Center for Informatics and Standards, ADA for review of ANSI/ADA and ISO standards administration information. Anita Mark, Senior Scientific Content Specialist, Evidence Synthesis and Translation Research, ADA SRI for editorial assistance. The mention of commercial products, their sources, or their use in connection with material reported herein is not to be construed as either an actual or implied endorsement of such products by the American Dental Association.

CONFLICTS OF INTEREST

The author has no conflicts of interest to report.

REFERENCES

1. Cochrane Rexmond C. Measures for progress: a history of the National Bureau of Standards. Washington, D: National Bureau of Standards, U.S. Department of Commerce; 1966.
2. Schooley James F. Responding to national needs: the national bureau of standards becomes the national institute of standards and technology, NIST SP 955. Washington, DC: U.S. Government Printing Office; 2000. p. 1032.
3. Dental products: standards, technical specification and technical reports. Available at: https://www.ada.org/resources/practice/dental-standards/standards-committee-on-dental-products/products-standards-technical-specifications-and-technical-reports. Accessed February 1, 2022.
4. ADA Standards Committee on Dental Products (SCDP). Available at: https://www.ada.org/resources/practice/dental-standards/standards-committee-on-dental-products. Accessed February 1, 2022.
5. Schmalz G, Jakubovics N, Schwendicke F. Normative approaches for oral health: standards, specifications, and guidelines. J Dent Res 2021. https://doi.org/10.1177/00220345211049695.
6. Stanford J. DMG Involvement in the Specification Program. In: Dental Materials Group governance. Available at: http://www-personal.umich.edu/~sbayne/DMG/000-Index-Files/index-DMG-frames.htm. Accessed February 1, 2022.
7. ISO/TC 106 Dentistry. In: ISO. Available at: https://committee.iso.org/home/tc106. Accessed January 19, 2022.
8. ADA Standards Program: Ensuring quality products for dentistry. American Dental Association, Chicago (IL). Available through ADA Center for Informatics and Standards, standards@ada.org.
9. U.S. TAG for ISO/TC 106 Dentistry. American Dental Association, Chicago (IL). Available through ADA Center for Informatics and Standards, standards@ada.org.
10. U.S. Representation in ISO. ANSI. Available at: https://www.ansi.org/iso/ansi-activities/us-tags. Accessed January 28, 2022.
11. ANSI History. ANSI. Available at: https://www.ansi.org/about/history. Accessed January 25, 2022.
12. Introduction: What is an ANS? In: ANSI. Available at: https://www.ansi.org/american-national-standards/ans-introduction/overview#introduction. Accessed January 25, 2022.

13. ANSI, Approval of American National Standards. Step 4: Consensus Body Voting. ANSI. Available at: https://www.ansi.org/american-national-standards/info-for-standards-developers/ans-approval/steps/step-4#: ~ :text=Consensus%20is%20demonstrated%2C%20in%20part,vote%20of%20the%20consensus%20body.&text=When%20recorded%20votes%20are%20taken,do%20so%20by%20the%20voter. Accessed February 1, 2022.

14. American Dental Association. *Technical Report: The consequence of changing from vertical to horizontal standards.* Chicago (IL): American Dental Association; 2003.

15. American Dental Association. *Technical Report: A road map to performance standards.* Chicago (IL): American Dental Association; 2007.

16. Jones D. Dental standards: fifty years of development. Br Dent J 2012;213:293–5. https://doi.org/10.1038/sj.bdj.2012.835.

17. Dentists' desk reference: materials, Instruments and equipment. 2nd edition. Chicago (IL): American Dental Association; 1983.

18. Megremis SM, Carey C. Corrosion and Tarnish of dental alloys. In: Cramer Stephen D, Covino Bernard S Jr, editors. ASM handbook, volume 13C corrosion: environments and industries13C. Materials Park (OH): ASM International; 2006. p. 891–921. Available at: https://www.nist.gov/publications/corrosion-and-tarnish-dental-alloys.

19. Revised ANSI/ADA Specification No. 5 for Dental Casting Alloys. JADA 1989; 18:379.

20. American National Standards Institute/American Dental Association. Specification No. 5 *Dental casting gold alloy.* Chicago (IL): American Dental Association Council on Scientific Affairs; 1989.

21. American National Standards Institute/American Dental Association. Specification No. 5 *Dental casting gold alloy.* Chicago (IL): American Dental Association Council on Scientific Affairs; 1998.

22. American National Standards/American Dental Association. Standard No. 134 *Metallic materials for fixed and removable restorations and appliances.* Chicago (IL): American Dental Association; 2013.

23. International Organization for Standardization. ISO 22674 *Dentistry – Metallic materials for fixed and removable restorations and appliances*, first edition, Geneva (Switzerland), 2006.

24. International Organization for Standardization. ISO/FDIS 22674 Dentistry – metallic materials for fixed and removable restorations and appliances, third edition, Geneva (Switzerland), 2022.

25. Price RB, Ferracane JL, Darvell BW, et al. Caveat emptor when purchasing dental products online. JADA 2022;153(Issue 3):P196–9. https://doi.org/10.1016/j.adaj.2021.10.013.

26. Technical Committees. ISO/TC 106 Dentistry. In: ISO. Available at: https://www.iso.org/committee/51218.html. Accessed January 19, 2022.

27. American National Standards/American Dental Association. Standard No.134 *Metallic materials for fixed and removable restorations and appliances.* Chicago (IL): American Dental Association; 2018.

28. International Organization for Standardization. ISO 22674 *Dentistry – metallic materials for fixed and removable restorations and appliances*, second edition, Geneva (Switzerland), 2016.

29. International Organization for Standardization. ISO 4049 *Dentistry – polymer-based restorative materials, third edition*, Geneva (Switzerland), 2000.

30. American National Standards/American Dental Association. Standard No. 27 *Direct filling resins*. Chicago (IL): American Dental Association; 1993.

31. American National Standards/American Dental Association. Standard No. 27 *Polymer-based restorative materials*. Chicago: American Dental Association; 2016.

32. International Organization for Standardization. ISO 4049 Dentistry – Polymer-based restorative materials, 5th edition, Geneva (Switzerland), 2019.

33. American National Standards/American Dental Association. Standard No. 27 *Polymer-based restorative materials*. Chicago (IL): American Dental Association; 2022.

34. Paffenbarger GC, Rupp NW. A history of the International Association for Dental Research Wilmer Souder Award in Dental Materials, with a short biography of Wilmer Souder. Dent Mater 1986;2(2):49–52.

35. Food and Drug Administration Modernization Act (FDAM) of 1997. FDA. Available at: https://www.fda.gov/regulatory-information/selected-amendments-fdc-act/food-and-drug-administration-modernization-act-fdama-1997. Accessed February 2, 2022.

36. Code of Federal Regulations, Title 21, Chapter 1, Subchapter H, Part 872. In: FDA. Available at: https://www.ecfr.gov/current/title-21/chapter-I/subchapter-H/part-872. Accessed January 27, 2022.

37. Appropriate Use of Voluntary Consensus Standards in Premarket Submissions for Medical Devices: Guidance for Industry and Food and Drug Administration Staff. FDA. Available at: https://www.fda.gov/regulatory-information/search-fda-guidance-documents/appropriate-use-voluntary-consensus-standards-premarket-submissions-medical-devices. Accessed February 2, 2022.

38. FDA Recognized Consensus Standards Database. FDA. Available at: https://www.accessdata.fda.gov/scripts/cdrh/cfdocs/cfstandards/search.cfm. Accessed February 2, 2022.

39. CDRH Learn: How to Study and Market Your Device: Standards, Module 4: How to Use Consensus Standards in Premarket Submissions. FDA. Available at: https://www.fda.gov/media/147787/download. Accessed February 2, 2022.

40. 510(k) Premarket Notification Database. FDA. Available at: https://www.accessdata.fda.gov/scripts/cdrh/cfdocs/cfPMN/pmn.cfm. Accessed February 2, 2022.

41. A History of Medical Device Regulation & Oversight in the United States. FDA. Available at: https://www.fda.gov/medical-devices/overview-device-regulation/history-medical-device-regulation-oversight-united-states. Accessed February 2, 2022.

42. U.S. Food and Drug Administration. Reporting Unlawful Sales of Medical Products on the Internet. FDA. Available at: https://www.accessdata.fda.gov/scripts/email/oc/buyonline/english.cfm. Accessed February 2, 2022.

43. MedWatch. The FDA safety information and adverse event reporting program. FDA. Available at: https://www.accessdata.fda.gov/scripts/medwatch/. Accessed February 2, 2022.

44. Price RBT. Light Curing in Dentistry. Dent Clin North Am 2017;61(4):751–78.

45. Megremis S, Ong V, Lukic H, et al. An ADA laboratory evaluation of light-emitting diode curing units. JADA 2014;145(11):1164–6.

46. An ADA Laboratory Evaluation of Light-Emitting Diode Curing Lights, ADA Professional Product Review. ADA 2014;9(Issue 4).

47. International Organization for Standardization. ISO 10650 Dentistry – *Powered polymerization activators*, 2nd edition, Geneva (Switzerland), 2018.

48. American National Standards/American Dental Association. Standard No. 48 *Curing lights (powered polymerization activators)*. Chicago (IL): American Dental Association; 2020.

49. 3M ESPE. Filtek Supreme Ultra Universal Restorative: Instructions for Use. St. Paul, MN: 3M ESPE. Available at: https://multimedia.3m.com/mws/media/6036220/3m-filtek-supreme-ultra-universal-restorative-instructions.pdf. Accessed February 1, 2022.

50. Ivoclar Vivadnet. Heliomolar: Instructions for Use – Light-curing resin-based dental restorative material. Rev.4, Jan. 29, 2018. Schaan, Liechtenstein: Ivoclar Vivadent. Available at: https://www.ivoclar.com/en_US/downloadcenter/?dc=us&lang=en#search-info-212=106139%2C1&details=21656. Accessed February 1, 2022.

UNITED STATES POSTAL SERVICE ® Statement of Ownership, Management, and Circulation (All Periodicals Publications Except Requester Publications)

1. Publication Title	2. Publication Number	3. Filing Date
DENTAL CLINICS OF NORTH AMERICA	566 – 480	9/18/2022

4. Issue Frequency	5. Number of Issues Published Annually	6. Annual Subscription Price
JAN, APR, JUL, OCT	4	$323.00

7. Complete Mailing Address of Known Office of Publication (Not printer) (Street, city, county, state, and ZIP+4®)

ELSEVIER INC.
230 Park Avenue, Suite 800
New York, NY 10169

Contact Person
Malathi Samayan

Telephone (Include area code)
91-44-4299-4507

8. Complete Mailing Address of Headquarters or General Business Office of Publisher (Not printer)

ELSEVIER INC.
230 Park Avenue, Suite 800
New York, NY 10169

9. Full Names and Complete Mailing Addresses of Publisher, Editor, and Managing Editor (Do not leave blank)

Publisher (Name and complete mailing address)

DOLORES MELONI, ELSEVIER INC.
1600 JOHN F KENNEDY BLVD. SUITE 1800
PHILADELPHIA, PA 19103-2899

Editor (Name and complete mailing address)

JOHN VASSALLO, ELSEVIER INC.
1600 JOHN F KENNEDY BLVD. SUITE 1800
PHILADELPHIA, PA 19103-2899

Managing Editor (Name and complete mailing address)

PATRICK MANLEY, ELSEVIER INC.
1600 JOHN F KENNEDY BLVD. SUITE 1800
PHILADELPHIA, PA 19103-2899

10. Owner (Do not leave blank. If the publication is owned by a corporation, give the name and address of the corporation immediately followed by the names and addresses of all stockholders owning or holding 1 percent or more of the total amount of stock. If not owned by a corporation, give the names and addresses of the individual owners. If owned by a partnership or other unincorporated firm, give its name and address as well as those of each individual owner. If the publication is published by a nonprofit organization, give its name and address.)

Full Name	Complete Mailing Address
WHOLLY OWNED SUBSIDIARY OF REED/ELSEVIER, US HOLDINGS	1600 JOHN F KENNEDY BLVD. SUITE 1800 PHILADELPHIA, PA 19103-2899

11. Known Bondholders, Mortgagees, and Other Security Holders Owning or Holding 1 Percent or More of Total Amount of Bonds, Mortgages, or Other Securities. If none, check box ► ☐ None

Full Name	Complete Mailing Address
N/A	

12. Tax Status (For completion by nonprofit organizations authorized to mail at nonprofit rates) (Check one)
The purpose, function, and nonprofit status of this organization and the exempt status for federal income tax purposes:
☒ Has Not Changed During Preceding 12 Months
☐ Has Changed During Preceding 12 Months (Publisher must submit explanation of change with this statement)

PS Form 3526, July 2014 [Page 1 of 4 (see instructions page 4)] PSN: 7530-01-000-9931   PRIVACY NOTICE: See our privacy policy on www.usps.com

---

13. Publication Title	14. Issue Date for Circulation Data Below
DENTAL CLINICS OF NORTH AMERICA	JULY 2022

15. Extent and Nature of Circulation			Average No. Copies Each Issue During Preceding 12 Months	No. Copies of Single Issue Published Nearest to Filing Date
a. Total Number of Copies (Net press run)			250	226
b. Paid Circulation (By Mail and Outside the Mail)	(1)	Mailed Outside-County Paid Subscriptions Stated on PS Form 3541 (Include paid distribution above nominal rate, advertiser's proof copies, and exchange copies)	140	125
	(2)	Mailed In-County Paid Subscriptions Stated on PS Form 3541 (Include paid distribution above nominal rate, advertiser's proof copies, and exchange copies)	0	0
	(3)	Paid Distribution Outside the Mails Including Sales Through Dealers and Carriers, Street Vendors, Counter Sales, and Other Paid Distribution Outside USPS®	87	62
	(4)	Paid Distribution by Other Classes of Mail Through the USPS (e.g., First-Class Mail®)	0	0
c. Total Paid Distribution (Sum of 15b (1), (2), (3), and (4))			227	187
d. Free or Nominal Rate Distribution (By Mail and Outside the Mail)	(1)	Free or Nominal Rate Outside-County Copies included on PS Form 3541	20	22
	(2)	Free or Nominal Rate In-County Copies Included on PS Form 3541	0	0
	(3)	Free or Nominal Rate Copies Mailed at Other Classes Through the USPS (e.g., First-Class Mail)	0	0
	(4)	Free or Nominal Rate Distribution Outside the Mail (Carriers or other means)	20	22
e. Total Free or Nominal Rate Distribution (Sum of 15d (1), (2), (3) and (4))			20	22
f. Total Distribution (Sum of 15c and 15e)			247	209
g. Copies not Distributed (See Instructions to Publishers #4 (page #3))			15	17
h. Total (Sum of 15f and g)			261	226
i. Percent Paid (15c divided by 15f times 100)			91.90%	89.47%

* If you are claiming electronic copies, go to line 16 on page 3. If you are not claiming electronic copies, skip to line 17 on page 3.

PS Form 3526, July 2014 (Page 2 of 4)

16. Electronic Copy Circulation	Average No. Copies Each Issue During Preceding 12 Months	No. Copies of Single Issue Published Nearest to Filing Date
a. Paid Electronic Copies		
b. Total Paid Print Copies (Line 15c) + Paid Electronic Copies (Line 16a)		
c. Total Print Distribution (Line 15f) + Paid Electronic Copies (Line 16a)		
d. Percent Paid (Both Print & Electronic Copies) (16b divided by 16c × 100)		

☒ I certify that 50% of all my distributed copies (electronic and print) are paid above a nominal price.

17. Publication of Statement of Ownership

☒ If the publication is a general publication, publication of this statement is required. Will be printed   ☐ Publication not required.
in the   OCTOBER 2022   issue of this publication.

18. Signature and Title of Editor, Publisher, Business Manager, or Owner

Malathi Samayan - Distribution Controller   *Malathi Samayan*   Date 9/18/2022

I certify that all information furnished on this form is true and complete. I understand that anyone who furnishes false or misleading information on this form or who omits material or information requested on the form may be subject to criminal sanctions (including fines and imprisonment) and/or civil sanctions (including civil penalties).

PS Form 3526, July 2014 (Page 3 of 4)   PRIVACY NOTICE: See our privacy policy on www.usps.com

Moving?

Make sure your subscription moves with you!

To notify us of your new address, find your **Clinics Account Number** (located on your mailing label above your name), and contact customer service at:

Email: journalscustomerservice-usa@elsevier.com

800-654-2452 (subscribers in the U.S. & Canada)
314-447-8871 (subscribers outside of the U.S. & Canada)

Fax number: 314-447-8029

Elsevier Health Sciences Division
Subscription Customer Service
3251 Riverport Lane
Maryland Heights, MO 63043

*To ensure uninterrupted delivery of your subscription, please notify us at least 4 weeks in advance of move.

Printed and bound by CPI Group (UK) Ltd, Croydon, CR0 4YY

19/10/2024

01776463-0001